ACSM'S

Fitness Assessment Manual

Sixth Edition

EDITORS

Yuri Feito, PhD, FACSM,
ACSM-CEP, EIM3

Education and Professional Development Strategist
American College of Sports Medicine
Indianapolis, Indiana

Meir Magal, PhD, FACSM,
ACSM-CEP

Chair, School of Mathematics and Sciences
Department of Exercise Science
Professor of Exercise Science
North Carolina Wesleyan College
Rocky Mount, North Carolina

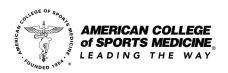

AMERICAN COLLEGE
of SPORTS MEDICINE
LEADING THE WAY®

ACSM'S
Fitness Assessment Manual

Sixth Edition

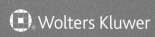

Philadelphia • Baltimore • New York • London
Buenos Aires • Hong Kong • Sydney • Tokyo

Acquisitions Editor: Lindsey Porambo
Senior Development Editor: Amy Millholen
Senior Editorial Coordinator: Lindsay Ries
Marketing Manager: Phyllis Hitner
Production Project Manager: Catherine Ott
Design Coordinator: Stephen Druding
Manufacturing Coordinator: Margie Orzech
Compositor: S4Carlisle Publishing Services
ACSM Publications Committee Chair: Jeffrey Potteiger, PhD, FACSM
ACSM Certification-Related Content Advisory Committee Chair: Dierdra Bycura, EdD, ACSM-CPT, ACSM-EP
ACSM Chief Operating Officer: Katie Feltman
ACSM Development Editor: Angela Chastain

Sixth Edition

9 8 7 6 5 4 3 2

Printed in Singapore

Library of Congress Cataloging-in-Publication Data

ISBN-13: 978-1-9751-6445-4

ISBN-10: 1-975164-45-8

Cataloging-in-Publication data available on request from the Publisher.

shop.lww.com

MKO822

Preface

The American College of Sports Medicine has long been a leader in advocating the health benefits associated with a physically active lifestyle. Clinicians, public health professionals, and allied health/fitness professionals can all provide tremendous benefit to their patients, communities, and clients with the expertise and knowledge of how to prescribe physical activity/exercise and how to subsequently measure the effects of these prescriptions. This *Manual* serves as the ideal text for all laboratory based fitness assessment courses in exercise science, physical therapy, and other health-related courses. Most users with a basic understanding of anatomy, physiology, and exercise physiology can find value in this *Manual* and likely realize that it will become a critical go-to text for the assessment laboratory.

As stated in Chapter 1 of this *Manual*, *physical fitness is the measurable outcome of a person's physical activity and exercise habits*. Thus, it is essential that exercise and health professionals are well versed in the methods of physical fitness assessment outcomes and interpretations with respect to body composition, cardiorespiratory fitness, muscular strength and endurance, and flexibility.

This sixth edition of *ACSM's Fitness Assessment Manual* provides important updates consistent with the most current resource information available on measuring physical fitness, and the *Manual's* intent remains to provide a comprehensive overview of why and how to perform assessments on the main components of physical fitness. New to this edition are chapters on metabolic calculations and electrocardiography. This *Manual* is an extension of assessment principles covered in the *ACSM's Guidelines for Exercise Testing and Prescription, Eleventh Edition* and includes many of the summary tables and figures from the *Guidelines*. After mastering the assessment procedures, the users of this *Manual* are encouraged to interpret the results with a clear understanding of the specific methodological limitations that exist for some of the procedures.

The value of physical fitness assessment results as a key health indicator is well accepted. Therefore, this *Manual* provides the foundational key concepts and methods of physical fitness assessment for all exercise science and allied health professionals so that each can continue to provide valid and reliable outcome measures to their respective populations.

FEATURES

- Reorganized and expanded information, including discussion of unique assessment principles and the major limitations of some assessment methods.
- Two new chapters: Metabolic Calculations (Chapter 6) and Electrocardiography (Chapter 9).
- Step-by-step instructions for assessment of physical fitness components and resources for interpretation of test results.
- Updated references to *ACSM's Guidelines for Exercise Testing and Prescription, Eleventh Edition*.
- More than 100 boxes, tables, and figures to help the reader understand the concepts of health-related physical fitness.

SUPPLEMENTAL MATERIALS

Supplemental materials for students and instructors are available at http://thepoint.lww.com/activate. Instructors can access the following:

- Test Bank
- PowerPoints
- Image Bank, including all figures and tables from the text
- Data Collection Forms

Students have access to the Data Collection Forms.

Acknowledgments

There are many individuals we would like to thank for without them this project would not have been possible. We would like to thank and acknowledge the tremendous work of all the previous editors of the *ACSM's Fitness Assessment Manual* and their vision and recognition for the need for a comprehensive manual of fitness assessment: Dr. Greg Dwyer, Dr. Shala Davis, Dr. Lenny Kaminsky, and Dr. Gary Liguori. We would like to thank the American College of Sports Medicine (ACSM) Certification-Related Content Advisory Committee and the Publications Committee for affording us the opportunity to work on this title, in particular, Drs. Dierdra Bycura and Jeff Potteiger. A special thanks go to Katie Feltman, *ACSM chief operating officer*, and Angela Chastain, *ACSM development editor*, for their time, dedication, and ongoing and unwavering support. Lastly, we also would like to recognize and express our appreciation and sincere gratitude to all the reviewers; without their dedicated work, this project would not have been possible.

We would like to dedicate this work to the ACSM Committee on Certification and Registry Boards (CCRB) and the Certification Department, past and present members and officers, for their selfless commitment to the profession and their diligent work on behalf of and for all ACSM certified professionals.

From Yuri Feito: It is said that a person's success is the product of those around them. As a result, I am indebted to the many professionals who have provided guidance and mentorships over the years, specifically Dr. NiCole Keith, Dr. Walt Thompson, Dr. Gary Liguori, and Dr. Deb Riebe; thank you for providing unwavering support, rich opportunities for professional growth, and invaluable friendships.

To my parents, Ana Maria and Fernando Feito, who gave everything up and emigrated multiple times, so that I could have the opportunities afforded by the "American Dream." To my brother, Ivan Feito, thank you for providing a guiding light. Lastly, to my wife and daughter, Kaitlin and Tatiana Nicole, thank you for your patience, encouragement, and support that made this work possible.

From Meir Magal: Over the years, my professional career has been influenced by a number of collaborative, honest, and passionate colleagues who have inspired me to pursue many opportunities, including the work on this ACSM book title. I would like to thank Dr. Deb Riebe, Dr. Greg Dwyer, and Dr. Walt Thompson — your unparallel support and insightful suggestions are invaluable.

Finally, I would like to thank my parents, Esther and Daniel Magal, for the values and ethics they have installed in me and also my wife Dana and my children, Yuval and Amit, for giving me the inspiration, support, and patience needed to complete this work.

Reviewers

Kevin D. Ballard, PhD, FACSM
Miami University
Oxford, Ohio

Daniel L. Carl, PhD, FACSM
University of Cincinnati
Cincinnati, Ohio

Julie M. Cousins, PhD
Albion University
Albion, Michigan

Amanda L. Zaleski, PhD
University of Connecticut
Storrs, Connecticut

Contents

Introduction

DEFINING PHYSICAL FITNESS

The purpose of the *American College of Sports Medicine's (ACSM) Fitness Assessment Manual* (FAM) is to introduce the exercise professional to the process of assessing physical fitness attributes and provide a thorough overview of the various tools and assessments one may use. Physical fitness is an umbrella term and is defined as a set of attributes or characteristics individuals have or achieve that relate to their ability to perform physical activity and activities of daily living (1). Physical fitness is divided into two subgroups: health-related physical fitness and sport- or skill-related physical fitness (Table 1.1).

TABLE 1.1 • Key Definitions Related to Physical Fitness[a]

Term	Definition
Physical activity	"Any bodily movement produced by the contraction of skeletal muscles that results in an increase in caloric requirements over resting energy expenditure"
Exercise	"A type of PA consisting of planned, structured, and repetitive bodily movement done to improve and/or maintain one or more components of physical fitness"
Physical fitness	"Set of attributes or characteristics individuals have or achieve that relate to their ability to perform PA and activities of daily living"
Health-related physical fitness	"Components more important to public health"
Skill-related physical fitness	Agility, balance, coordination, power, speed, and reaction time, "Components related to athletic ability"

[a]Source for definitions from Reference (2).

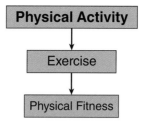

Figure 1.1 Relationships between physical activity and its subcomponents.

Whereas the latter is more related to sport performance, as the name implies, the former consists of specific components of physical fitness that are often linked to public health (1). Through the process of exercise prescription, the exercise professional should be aware that these components may not be exclusive (health related or skill related), and with some populations such as older adults, some of the sport/skill attributes may also be important for health (2).

By definition, physical fitness has considerable overlap with exercise and physical activity (PA), often leading to a misuse of the terms because of their interrelated nature. Instead, the exercise professional should be able to distinguish each term and apply them in the proper context (see Table 1.1).

PA has been shown to have a linear relationship to health and therefore is a term that must be clearly defined and understood. *Physical activity* is defined as "any bodily movement produced by the contraction of skeletal muscles that results in an increase in caloric requirements over resting energy expenditure" (1). Exercise, a form of PA, is more specific and is defined as planned, structured, repetitive, and purposive, in the sense that improvement or maintenance of one or more components of physical fitness is the objective (1).

To achieve physical fitness, an individual must engage in exercise. Exercise can then be specific to the participants' goals — either for health or for performance (see Figure 1.1). Although this manual provides the means of assessing several components of fitness, the *ACSM's Guidelines for Exercise Testing and Prescription, Eleventh Edition* (*GETP11*) provides specific guidelines for exercise training.

Ultimately, physical fitness is a measurable set of characteristics largely determined by the PA habits of an individual. Although genetics also plays a role in the level of physical fitness one can achieve, those with the highest levels of physical fitness tend to have maximized their exercise training.

Components of Physical Fitness

ACSM has been a leader in setting guidelines for the assessment of physical fitness. Five measurable components of physical fitness are depicted in Figure 1.2.

Cardiorespiratory endurance refers to the ability of the circulatory and respiratory systems to supply oxygen during sustained PA. **Cardiorespiratory fitness** is related to the ability to perform large-muscle, dynamic, moderate- to high-intensity exercise for prolonged periods of time. The methods of assessment of cardiorespiratory fitness are provided in Chapters 4 and 5 of this manual.

Body composition refers to the relative amount or percentage of different types of body tissue (bone, fat, muscle) that are related to health. The most common health-related measure is that of total body fat percentage; however, it should be noted that there are no established criterion values for this measure related to health parameters. The methods used to assess body composition are provided in Chapter 3 of this manual.

Muscular strength and *muscular endurance*, although two separate components of physical fitness, are often combined into one component termed "muscular fitness."

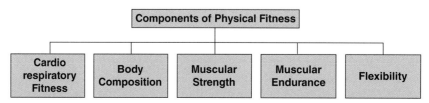

Figure 1.2 Physical fitness is not a single entity but rather a sum of five measurable components.

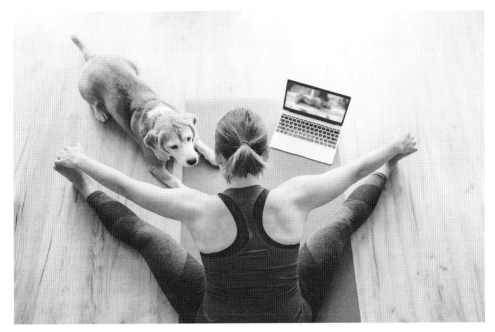

Figure 1.3 Flexibility is one of the components of physical fitness.

Muscular strength is the ability of a muscle group to develop maximal contractile force against a resistance in a single contraction and is related to the ability to perform activities that require high levels of muscular force.

Muscular endurance is the ability of a muscle group to execute repeated contractions over a period of time sufficient to cause muscular fatigue or to maintain a specific percentage of the maximum voluntary contraction for a prolonged period of time. Chapter 7 of this manual has specific measurement information on muscular endurance.

Flexibility is the ability to move a joint through its complete range of movement. Chapter 8 of this manual has specific measurement information on flexibility. Figure 1.3 displays one type of assessment of flexibility.

Even though an individual's appearance or exercise habits may be viewed as evidence of physical fitness and/or health, these can be very misleading "criteria." Instead, because one single measure of physical fitness, or health, does not currently exist, there is a need to have a battery of valid and reliable assessments. It is not uncommon for regular exercisers to spend most of their time training only one component of physical fitness, for example, frequent long-distance running. This person, who may appear to be thin, is also often considered "physically fit" and, indeed, maybe in terms of cardiorespiratory fitness alone. However, this person is also likely below average in terms of muscular strength and flexibility. Likewise, someone who performs high levels of resistance training as the sole form of exercise may appear to be quite muscular and viewed as physically fit and, indeed, maybe in terms of muscular fitness (strength and endurance). However, similar to the person who runs a lot, this person is also likely to be below average in certain areas of fitness, including cardiorespiratory fitness and flexibility. Thus, it is important to view physical fitness as an integration of multiple components.

IMPORTANCE OF MEASURING PHYSICAL FITNESS

Relationship of Physical Fitness to Health

Throughout history, humans have broadly recognized the relationship between physical fitness and health. In ancient China, records of organized exercise as a means of health promotion date from 2500 B.C., and there is much evidence that the ancient Greeks "emphasized the importance of physical well-being, fitness, and a healthy lifestyle" (3). Yet systematic investigation and research of this relationship did not begin until the early 1900s, and from that time forward, scientific literature has firmly established the relationship between PA and health.

In 1996, the U.S. Surgeon General Report (SGR) released the *Physical Activity and Health* report (4), which provided an extensive review of research demonstrating various health benefits obtained from

---

Box 1.1	Some Benefits of Regular Physical Activity and/or Exercise

Improvement in Cardiovascular and Respiratory Function
- Increased maximal oxygen uptake, resulting from both central and peripheral adaptations
- Decreased heart rate and blood pressure at a given submaximal intensity

Reduction in Cardiovascular Disease Risk Factors
- Reduced resting systolic/diastolic pressures
- Increased serum high-density lipoprotein cholesterol and decreased serum triglycerides

Decreased Morbidity and Mortality
- Higher activity and/or fitness levels are associated with lower incidence rates for combined cardiovascular diseases, coronary artery disease, stroke, and many other chronic diseases.

Other Benefits
- Decreased anxiety and depression
- Improved cognitive function

PA. The SGR also emphasized what is termed the *dose–response* relationship, where *dose* refers to the amount of PA and/or exercise, and *response* refers to the resultant health outcome. Although the evidence is quite clear that exercise doses result in many health benefits (as noted in Box 1.1), the exact minimal dose of PA and/or exercise required to produce health benefits was not yet clearly discerned.

The 2008 *Physical Activity Guidelines for Americans* (5) and more recently the *2018 (second edition) Physical Activity Guidelines for Americans* (6) represent the latest comprehensive report based on major research findings regarding the relationship between PA and health. The *2018 Guidelines* is an essential resource for all exercise professionals and provides the following summary suggestions regarding duration and intensity of PA for adults:

- Adults should move more and sit less throughout the day. Some PA is better than none. Adults who sit less and do any amount of moderate-to-vigorous PA gain some health benefits.
- For substantial health benefits, adults should do at least 150 to 300 min · wk^{-1} of moderate-intensity, or 75 to 150 min · wk^{-1} of vigorous-intensity aerobic PA, or an equivalent combination of moderate- and vigorous-intensity aerobic activity. Preferably, aerobic activity should be spread throughout the week.
- Additional health benefits are gained by engaging in PA beyond the equivalent of 300 minutes of moderate-intensity PA a week.
- Adults should also do muscle-strengthening activities of moderate or greater intensity and that involve all major muscle groups on 2 or more d · wk^{-1}, because these activities provide additional health benefits.

In addition, the recently published second edition of the *Physical Activity Guidelines for Americans* clearly supports the numerous health benefits resulting from regular participation in PA and structured exercise programs (6). Given that it is PA and exercise that promote the maintenance or improvement in physical fitness, and physical fitness is the measurable outcome of a person's PA and exercise habits, therein lies a need for measuring these components. The following are among some important reasons for assessing physical fitness:

- *Educating participants about their present fitness status relative to health-related standards and age- and sex-matched norms.* Good health care for an individual includes knowing important personal health-related information, such as one's cholesterol level and blood pressure. Similarly, knowledge of fitness measurements would support optimizing personal health.
- *Providing data that are helpful in the development of individualized exercise prescriptions to address all health/fitness components.* Maintenance or improvement in the different components of fitness requires different types of exercise training. Thus, although there are some generalized exercise recommendations for good health, the exercise prescription can and should be tailored to the specific needs and goals of the individual. This is best achieved by having current fitness measurements.
- *Collecting baseline and follow-up data that allow evaluation of progress by exercise program participants.* Other personal health information, such as cholesterol and blood pressure, is tracked over

time. Similarly, measuring fitness components periodically can aid an individual in managing personal health. Measurements through time can also help identify whether training program modifications need to be made to improve some components, while maintaining desired levels of the other components.

- *Motivating participants by establishing reasonable and attainable fitness goals.* Knowing one's fitness measures provides a baseline for individualizing a physical fitness program and is also a key starting point to motivate change. Fitness goals can be based on these initial assessments and followed periodically with reassessments, allowing for short-term positive feedback, which is a strong motivator to positive change.

Relationship of Physical Fitness to Function

It has been well recognized that many aspects of sport performance are related to physical fitness. Indeed, there are several sport-related physical fitness components, such as power, agility, and balance, that may affect health and can be assessed. For example, power training may affect balance, which, in turn, will reduce falls (7). Although not necessarily related to a specific performance outcome, the components of fitness are now being recognized as important to the function of everyday tasks and leisure-time pursuits. For example, completing the basic tasks of everyday living, also known as activities of daily living (ADLs), requires an individual functional capacity of about 5.0 metabolic equivalents (METs). However, this does not reflect a particularly high level of physical fitness and only represents the ability to manage minimal household tasks. To engage in leisure-time pursuits, which could range from backyard landscaping to family ice skating or a weekend camping trip, sufficient levels of each of the components of fitness will be necessary.

These are only examples of how fitness is related to function. Certainly, the ability to perform basic daily functions and also to enjoy leisure-time pursuits depends on one's physical fitness level, and this becomes even more apparent as one ages. Figure 1.4 shows an example of a recreational activity that can be performed throughout one's lifetime if adequate levels of fitness are maintained.

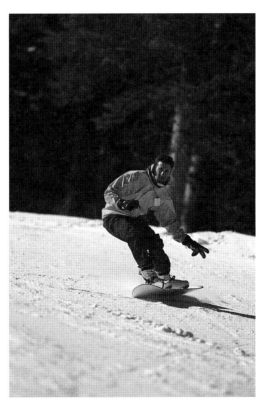

Figure 1.4 People who are physically fit are capable of performing both occupational and recreational activities throughout their lifetimes.

FUNDAMENTAL PRINCIPLES OF ASSESSMENT

For each of the components of fitness, there are various assessment methods that can be used. This manual provides an overview of assessment procedures and interpretations for each fitness component. However, regardless of which component is assessed, there are fundamental principles that should be applied in performing physical fitness assessments.

A Specific Assessment Objective

A clear purpose should be identified prior to performing any assessment. A list of important reasons for performing fitness measurements was provided earlier. Both the participant and the exercise professional should have a clear understanding of the objective of the assessment. Knowing this objective will ensure the selection of the most appropriate procedure.

The Gold Standard (True Measure)

A general principle in assessment is that one test is considered the criterion test or gold standard, that is, it is considered the definitive or true measure. This does not necessarily mean that it is a perfect test, but that given the current state of information, it is considered the best test that exists for measuring a specific variable. Although ideal, the gold standard test may not always be used owing to several different circumstances, such as the need for expensive equipment, specially trained personnel, the requirement of extensive time, or the increased risk level to the participant.

Error of Measurement

If the use of the gold standard test is not feasible, other tests can be employed to estimate the variable of interest; however, this typically leads to some level of inaccuracy. For most physiologic variables, such as measures of fitness, the distribution of errors in measurement follows that of the normal bell curve, as depicted in Figure 1.5. When expressing a measurement value from an estimation-type test, the value should include the error range. This is typically expressed as ± 1 standard deviation from the mean or, in prediction equations, the standard error of estimate (SEE). For example, if a test reported a mean value of 50 with a standard deviation of 5 (50 ± 5), this means that if there were 100 cases with a value estimated to be 50, 68 of those cases would have an actual value between 45 and 55, 95 of the cases would have an actual value between 40 and 60, and 5 cases would have values either <40 or >60. Specifics about measurement errors for different fitness tests are provided in future chapters in this text. Thus, it is essential for the exercise professional to understand the amount of error in measurement when using indirect tests to estimate a fitness component.

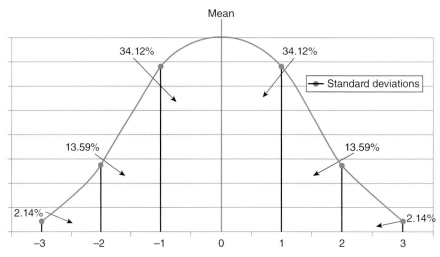

Figure 1.5 Characteristics of the normal bell curve.

Equipment Calibration

Some instruments or equipment employed in assessments provide accurate measurements every time if used correctly. For example, a wall-mounted stadiometer is a stable device that measures height accurately. However, over time, a device such as a weight scale may produce variable readings for standard weight. To ensure the accuracy of the reading, the device must be calibrated prior to the testing session and properly adjusted to produce an accurate reading.

Standardization

Another fundamental principle for assessment involves following standardized procedures. Many factors can cause variability in a measurement, so applying uniform standards reduces or eliminates the sources of variability. These may include pretest instructions that may extend to 24 hours prior to the test (*e.g.*, no vigorous exercise on the day prior to the test) and the environmental conditions of the fitness testing facility (*e.g.*, temperature between 20°C and 24°C).

Interpretation Issues

Ideally, there exists one standard that can be used to interpret the results of a test. For example, it is well accepted that in a health assessment that includes a total cholesterol measurement, the results are interpreted with the values established by the European Society of Cardiology/European Atherosclerosis Society (ESC/EAS), the American Association of Clinical Endocrinologists (AACE), and the American College of Endocrinology (ACE) (8,9). Unfortunately, no national set of standards has been established for assessment and interpretation of fitness components. In this text, some of the most commonly used tools for interpretation of results are provided.

Types of Standards

There are two basic types of standards: criterion referenced and normative. **Criterion-referenced standards** are a set of scores that classify the result as desirable (or above or below desirable) based on some external criteria, such as the betterment of health, and as determined by a group of experts. Criterion-referenced standards often use adjectives, such as "excellent" or "poor," in classifying test results. **Normative standards**, sometimes referred to as *norms*, are based on the past performance of groups of individuals with similar characteristics (*e.g.*, age, gender). Thus, with normative standards, a comparison is made between the participant's performance and the performance of similar individuals. The data interpretation classifications often use a percentile score, such as 90th and 50th. In fitness assessment, there are more normative standards than criterion-referenced standards available for interpretation. As mentioned in GETP11, the number of visible transgender individuals is increasing, and they are therefore more likely to be encountered by fitness and exercise professionals in their daily work. The current estimated number of adults reported as transgender in the United States is approximately 1.4 million (10). In regard to fitness testing and health risk status, many norms and criteria are based on sex recorded at birth, along with age and other discriminating factors. Herein lies the challenge to the exercise professional, as currently, there is little evidence to guide the decision as to which sex-based criteria and norms to use for transgender individuals undergoing medical treatment. Additionally, although it may seem intuitive to use the current gender identification to align with health and fitness norms, there is little current evidence to support this as of yet. Therefore, because there are few data and few norms for individuals in the midst of a medical treatment for gender incongruence, it may be best to use collected data only on an intrapersonal basis while norms are being developed.

THE EXERCISE PROFESSIONAL

Merriam-Webster defines a profession as "a calling requiring specialized knowledge and often long and intensive academic preparation" and a *professional* as one who "conforms to the technical and ethical standards of his or her profession" (11).

There are no universally defined professional standards for those who work with people in the areas of physical fitness or exercise. However, some states have pursued licensure legislation that would set standards for professionals that provide these services. In addition, some employers have voluntarily set standards for individuals they hire to perform physical fitness assessments or to supervise exercise programs.

Academic Training

For many years, universities have offered degrees focused on exercise, although the exact title of the degree (*e.g.*, exercise physiology, exercise science, kinesiology) and curriculum requirements are unique to the institution. Various exercise-related degrees are offered at the associate, bachelor, master, and doctoral levels, each requiring different expectations and outcomes. ACSM, along with other professional organizations, has initiated efforts to support accreditation of academic programs that offer degree programs in exercise science. The Committee on Accreditation for the Exercise Sciences (CoAES) was established in 2004 with the support of the Commission on Accreditation of Allied Health Education Programs (CAAHEP). Under CoAES, there are three levels of accreditations: (1) exercise physiology for master's degree awarding programs, (2) exercise science for bachelor's degree awarding programs, and (3) personal fitness training for associates degree awarding programs (12). Students graduating from an accredited program will have demonstrated proficiently in most if not all of the assessments found in this manual.

Credentials

Many people who work in the area of physical fitness assessment and/or who provide exercise program services obtain a certification, usually from a professional organization, which attests that they have achieved a minimum level of knowledge and/or competency. Although numerous different organizations and groups offer some form of certification related to physical fitness assessment and/or exercise services, ACSM has long been a leader in providing these types of certifications. The Institute for Credentialing Excellence created the National Commission for Certifying Agencies (NCCA) to demonstrate that certification programs have met minimal standards for professional competence. Presently, ACSM offers four different types of NCCA-accredited certifications, with a wide range of prerequisites needed to be able to sit for the different examinations (2,13). A detailed description of the three health fitness certifications and the one clinical certification can be found online at https://www.acsm.org/get-stay-certified/get-certified.

REFERENCES

1. Caspersen CJ, Powell KE, Christenson GM. Physical activity, exercise, and physical fitness: definitions and distinctions for health-related research. *Public Health Rep.* 1985;100(2):126–31.
2. ACSM. *ACSM's Guidelines for Exercise Testing and Prescription.* 11th ed. Philadelphia (PA): Wolters Kluwer; 2021.
3. MacAuley D. A history of physical activity, health and medicine. *J R Soc Med.* 1994;87(1):32–5.
4. U.S. Department of Health and Human Services. Physical activity and health: a report of the Surgeon General [Internet]. 1996 [cited 2020 January 21]. Available from: https://www.cdc.gov/nccdphp/sgr/pdf/execsumm.pdf.
5. Physical Activity Guidelines Advisory Committee. *Physical Activity Guidelines for Americans.* Washington (DC): US Department of Health and Human Services; 2008. p. 15–34; 76 pp.
6. U.S. Department of Health and Human Services. Physical Activity Guidelines for Americans [Internet]. 2nd ed. U.S. Department of Health and Human Services. 2018 [cited 2020 January 21]. Available from: https://health.gov/paguidelines/second-edition/pdf/Physical_Activity_Guidelines_2nd_edition.pdf.
7. Garber CE, Blissmer B, Deschenes MR, et al. Quantity and quality of exercise for developing and maintaining cardiorespiratory, musculoskeletal, and neuromotor fitness in apparently healthy adults: guidance for prescribing exercise. *Med Sci Sports Exerc.* 2011;43(7):1334–59.
8. Catapano AL, Graham I, De Backer G, et al. ESC/EAS guidelines for the management of dyslipidaemias. *Eur Heart J.* 2016;37(39):2999–3058.
9. Jellinger PS, Handelsman Y, Rosenblit PD, et al. American Association of Clinical Endocrinologists and American College of Endocrinology guidelines for management of dyslipidemia and prevention of cardiovascular disease. *Endocr Pract.* 2017;23(s2):1–87.
10. Flores AR, Herman JL, Gates GJ, Brown TNT. How many adults identify as transgender in the United States? [Internet]. Los Angeles (CA): The Williams Institute; 2016 [cited 2020 May 12]. Available from: https://williamsinstitute.law.ucla.edu/publications/trans-adults-united-states/
11. Merriam-Webster.com. Professional [Internet]. 2020 [cited 2020 January 21]. Available from: https://www.merriam-webster.com/dictionary/professional.
12. Committee on Accreditation for the Exercise Sciences. Standards and Guidelines [Internet]. 2020 [cited 2020 January 21]. Available from: http://www.coaes.org/.
13. Magal M, Neric FB. ACSM Certifications: defining an exercise profession from concept to assessment. *ACSM's Health Fit J.* 2020;24(*1*):12–18.

Preparticipation Health Screening and Evaluation

CHAPTER OUTLINE

RATIONALE FOR PREASSESSMENT SCREENING

Physical fitness assessment procedures range from those requiring no exercise to those in need of vigorous or even maximal physical exertion. The risk associated with conducting assessments can range from no risk at all to a serious risk to the individual. If the assessments are limited to nonexercise procedures posing no risk (*e.g.*, a skinfold measurement for body composition), there would be no need to perform a preassessment screening. However, because exercise-based assessments pose both cardiovascular (CV) and musculoskeletal injury (MSI) risks, a fitness assessment requiring exercise will also require a preassessment screening. The individual risks are related to both the intensity of the exercise and the activity habits of the client. The *American College of Sports Medicine's (ACSM) Guidelines for Exercise Testing and Prescription, Eleventh Edition (GETP11)* emphasizes this point stating, "the risk for activity-associated sudden cardiac death (SCD) and acute myocardial infarction (AMI) is known to be highest among those with underlying cardiovascular disease (CVD) who perform unaccustomed vigorous physical activity (PA)." More specific information about CVD risks associated with exercise can be found in *Chapter 1* of *ACSM's GETP11*, with summarized data about event rates found in tables 1.3 to 1.5. Similarly, the risk of MSIs are greater in those individuals with known musculoskeletal diseases, previous injuries, exercise intensity, the type of activity, as well as in those who are inactive. It is therefore critical to know the health and activity history of all individuals who will be performing fitness assessments involving exercise.

INFORMED CONSENT

The first step in the process of a fitness assessment is completion of the informed consent. Therefore, the first contact most individuals have with a program is with the person who administers the informed consent and conducts the risk screening. A client's impression of a program may thus depend on this first contact with the staff. Thinking about fitness testing may create anxiety in the client, and the test results may create other unpleasant feelings. Every effort should be made to help the client relax and focus on the beneficial information afforded from the results of the fitness assessment. Although the exact approach may vary somewhat depending on the client's personality, performing this initial stage of the assessment with calm professionalism is recommended.

The privacy of the client's health information is paramount and should be protected as described in the Health Insurance Portability and Accountability Act (HIPAA) (1,2). Completion of the informed consent must precede the health risk appraisal because determination of the health risk status will require the exchange of private health information and may require procedures that involve physical risk (*e.g.*, blood testing). In addition, if the fitness assessment requires exercise, there are risks involved.

The essential steps in executing the informed consent are the following:

- Explaining the purpose of the assessments
- Describing the procedures to be used
- Describing the risks and discomforts associated with the assessments
- Describing the benefits obtained from the assessments
- Describing alternatives (if any)
- Describing the responsibilities required of the client
- Encouraging the client to ask questions at any time
- Explaining how data will be handled (confidentiality)
- Explaining that the client can withdraw his or her consent and stop the assessment process at any time

An example of an informed consent form is provided in Box 2.1; however, there are many variations in informed consent available from different sources. All professionals performing fitness assessments should take time to find a standard form that closely matches a given facility's needs and assessments. Modifications to the form can be made to fit specific needs of the fitness assessment program, and it is recommended that legal counsel review the final form to limit the chances of legal liability. Finally, it is essential that different informed consent forms be used for each different component of a program (*i.e.*, assessments, exercise programs, and research projects).

Box 2.1	Sample of Informed Consent Form for a Symptom-Limited Exercise Test

Informed Consent for an Exercise Test

1. Purpose and Explanation of the Test

   You will perform an exercise test on a cycle ergometer or a motor-driven treadmill. The exercise intensity will begin at a low level and will be advanced in stages depending on your fitness level. We may stop the test at any time because of signs of fatigue or changes in your heart rate, electrocardiogram, or blood pressure or because of symptoms you may experience. It is important for you to realize that you may stop when you wish because of feelings of fatigue or any other discomfort.

2. Attendant Risks and Discomforts

   There exists the possibility of certain changes occurring during the test. These include abnormal blood pressure; fainting; irregular, fast, or slow heart rhythm; and, in rare instances, heart attack, stroke, or death. Every effort will be made to minimize these risks by evaluation of preliminary information relating to your health and fitness and by careful observations during testing. Emergency equipment and trained personnel are available to deal with unusual situations that may arise.

3. Responsibilities of the Participant

   Information you possess about your health status or previous experiences of heart-related symptoms (*e.g.*, shortness of breath with low-level activity; pain; pressure; tightness; heaviness in the chest, neck, jaw, back, and/or arms) with physical effort may affect the safety of your exercise test. Your prompt reporting of these and any other unusual feelings with effort during the exercise test itself is very important. You are responsible for fully disclosing your medical history as well as symptoms that may occur during the test. You are also expected to report all medications (including nonprescription) taken recently and, in particular, those taken today to the testing staff.

4. Benefits to Be Expected

   The results obtained from the exercise test may assist in the diagnosis of your illness, in evaluating the effect of your medications, or in evaluating what type of PAs you might do with low risk.

5. Inquiries

   Any questions about the procedures used in the exercise test or the results of your test are encouraged. If you have any concerns or questions, please ask us for further explanations.

6. Use of Medical Records

   The information that is obtained during exercise testing will be treated as privileged and confidential as described in the Health Insurance Portability and Accountability Act (HIPAA) of 1996. It is not to be released or revealed to any individual, except your referring physician, without your written consent. However, the information obtained may be used for statistical analysis or scientific purposes with your right to privacy retained.

7. Freedom of Consent

   I hereby consent to voluntarily engage in an exercise test to determine my exercise capacity and state of CV health. My permission to perform this exercise test is given voluntarily. I understand that I am free to stop the test at any point if I so desire.

   I have read this form, and I understand the test procedures that I will perform and the attendant risks and discomforts. Knowing these risks and discomforts, and having had an opportunity to ask questions that have been answered to my satisfaction, I consent to participate in this test.

_____   _____
Date   Signature of Patient/Participant

_____   _____
Date   Signature of Witness

_____   _____
Date   Signature of Physician or Authorized Delegate

The Informed Consent Process

The informed consent is not just a form requiring a signature; rather, it is a process of documentation that attests to the fact that a clear communication has taken place between the individual who is desiring to have the fitness assessment and the professional who will be administering the assessments. It is through the process of articulating the purposes, risks, and benefits of the assessment that professionals help their clients have the knowledge and understanding needed to make informed decisions about whether to complete the fitness assessment. Although the evidence suggests that for most people expected benefits of performing the assessment outweigh the associated risks, each client needs to make an informed decision on the basis of personal factors.

To begin the informed consent process, the client should carefully read the entire form or have the form read aloud while following along. Next, the professional should review some of the key elements of the assessment, including purpose, risks and benefits, and overview of procedures (Figure 2.1). One key point of emphasis is that the client will play an important role in the process. Specifically, the client has the responsibility of informing test administrators of any problems experienced (past, present, and during the physical fitness assessment) that may increase the risk of the test or preclude participation. This information is essential to minimize the risks involved with the assessment and can also optimize the benefits. Finally, the client should be allowed and encouraged to ask questions before signing the informed consent.

Explanation of Procedures

The professional should be prepared to provide a brief description of each assessment to be performed and answer client questions in detail. The following are examples of some common fitness assessments and sample explanations of each. Detailed reviews of all the fitness assessments are provided in Chapters 3, 4, 5, 7, and 8.

- Anthropometry or body composition: "This test is being performed to obtain an estimate of your total body fat percentage. We will determine your body fat percentage by taking measurements with a set of calipers at different sites on your body. We do this by pinching and pulling on the skin at these different locations. We will also measure some body girths with a tape measure to provide an indication of fat distribution on your body."
- Cardiorespiratory fitness: "This test is being performed to obtain an estimate of your cardiorespiratory fitness. The test will require you to exercise on a stationary cycle or a treadmill for 6 to 12 minutes. The intensity of the test will be limited to a level below your maximal exertion point. Your heart rate (HR) and blood pressure (BP) response will be monitored throughout the duration of the test."
- Flexibility: "Because range of motion (ROM) is joint specific, measuring the ROM of different joints by using a goniometer is necessary. The goniometer is similar to a protractor. We will place the goniometer at a given joint line by aligning the axis (pin) of the goniometer and your given joint's axis of rotation and measure the angle between the stabilizing and movement arms (measurement is expressed in degrees)."
- Muscular fitness: "Although there is no one test that can measure your total muscular fitness, this test is being performed to obtain a measure of your muscle strength by having you squeeze a hand grip dynamometer as hard as you can. We will also measure muscle endurance by having you perform as many push-ups as you can."

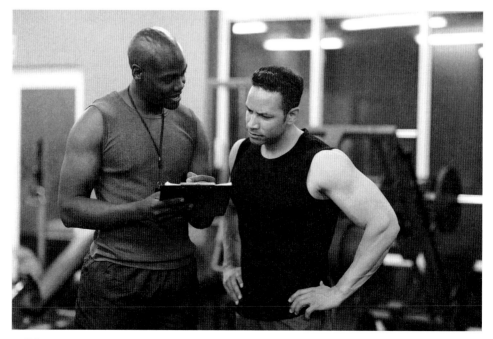

Figure 2.1 An important aspect of the informed consent process is reviewing key elements with the client and answering any questions the client may have.

EXERCISE PREPARTICIPATION HEALTH SCREENING

Exercise preparticipation health screening is the next step in the process of fitness assessment. An exercise professional should complete at least one of the following two processes: (a) ACSM exercise preparticipation health screening process (Figure 2.2) or (b) the Physical Activity Readiness Questionnaire for Everyone (PAR-Q+) (see Figure 2.4). The latter is often described as an alternative self-guided screener. Regardless of the chosen process, this information may be used for determining the individual's readiness to maintain or engage in PA.

ACSM Preparticipation Screening Algorithm

Chapter 2 of *ACSM's GETP11* provides a thorough overview of the exercise preparticipation health screening process. This process is designed to identify those individuals who may be at risk for adverse

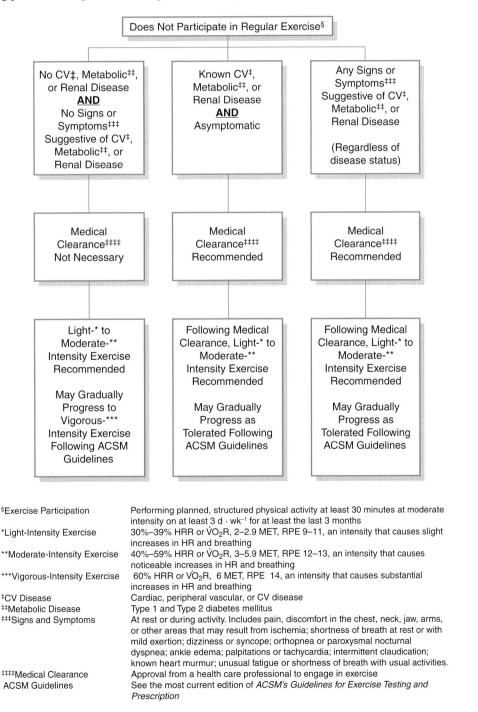

§Exercise Participation	Performing planned, structured physical activity at least 30 minutes at moderate intensity on at least 3 d · wk⁻¹ for at least the last 3 months	
*Light-Intensity Exercise	30%–39% HRR or V̇O₂R, 2–2.9 MET, RPE 9–11, an intensity that causes slight increases in HR and breathing	
**Moderate-Intensity Exercise	40%–59% HRR or V̇O₂R, 3–5.9 MET, RPE 12–13, an intensity that causes noticeable increases in HR and breathing	
***Vigorous-Intensity Exercise	60% HRR or V̇O₂R, 6 MET, RPE 14, an intensity that causes substantial increases in HR and breathing	
‡CV Disease	Cardiac, peripheral vascular, or CV disease	
‡‡Metabolic Disease	Type 1 and Type 2 diabetes mellitus	
‡‡‡Signs and Symptoms	At rest or during activity. Includes pain, discomfort in the chest, neck, jaw, arms, or other areas that may result from ischemia; shortness of breath at rest or with mild exertion; dizziness or syncope; orthopnea or paroxysmal nocturnal dyspnea; ankle edema; palpitations or tachycardia; intermittent claudication; known heart murmur; unusual fatigue or shortness of breath with usual activities.	
‡‡‡‡Medical Clearance	Approval from a health care professional to engage in exercise	
ACSM Guidelines	See the most current edition of *ACSM's Guidelines for Exercise Testing and Prescription*	

Figure 2.2 The Preparticipation Logic Model. ACSM, American College of Sports Medicine; CV, cardiovascular disease; HR, heart rate; HRR, heart rate reserve; RPE, rating of perceived exertion.

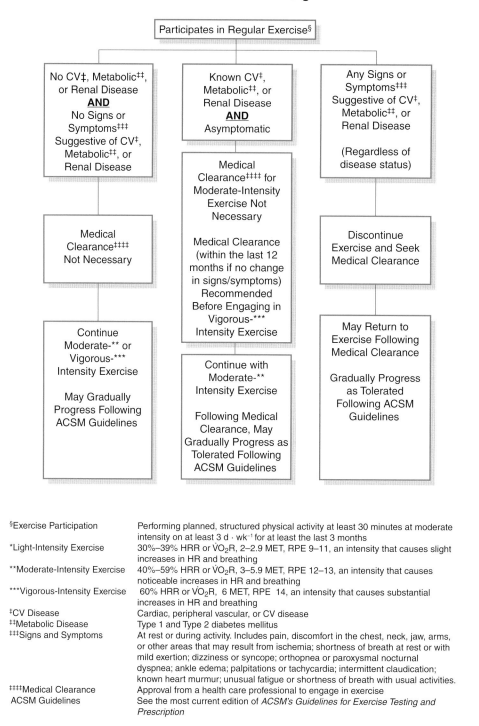

Figure 2.2 *(Continued)*

exercise-related CV events. ACSM supports the idea that regular PA is a key public health tool and that any preparticipation health screening process should be free of unwarranted barriers so that adopting a physically active lifestyle is attainable for all.

The algorithm-derived exercise preparticipation health screening, such as the informed consent, is a dynamic process and will vary in its scope and components depending on the client's health and medical status (*e.g.*, signs, symptoms, or previously diagnosed CV, metabolic, and/or renal diseases) and the PA or exercise program goals of the individual (*e.g.*, moderate intensity vs. vigorous intensity). In fact, there are several reasons why clients should be screened before involvement in a fitness assessment program, including:

- Determining the clients' current PA levels
- Determining the clients' PA goals

- Identifying clients who may present with signs and symptoms suggesting the presence of underlying CV, metabolic, and renal disease
- Identifying clients with diagnosed CV, metabolic, and/or renal disease
- Using the abovementioned information to make recommendations for preparticipation medical clearance

Signs or Symptoms Suggestive of Cardiopulmonary Disease

There are several visible signs or reported symptoms a client may have that would indicate the likelihood of having CV, metabolic, and/or renal disease. These signs and symptoms are listed in Table 2.1. If a client has any of the listed signs or symptoms, he or she should be immediately referred to a physician for follow-up and to obtain medical clearance before participation in any fitness assessments.

To make a decision about the presence or absence of a sign or symptom suggestive of CV, metabolic, or renal disease, the exercise professional should follow the specific criteria for each. Some key features that aid in clarifying whether the reported feeling should be designated as a symptom are listed in Table 2.1. For example, a client may report that he or she has experienced chest pain. The key features that classify this pain as *favoring an ischemic origin* are the *character* of the pain, the *location* of the pain, and the factors associated with *provoking* the pain. It is important to ask the client to describe the feeling with as little prompting for specific characteristics as possible. Ideally, the exercise professional may want the client to describe the feeling using self-selected words. Asking a client to describe the location of the pain is better than asking if there is pain in the shoulders, neck, or arms.

Using the Preparticipation Logic Model

ACSM, as outlined in *GETP11* (3), recommends that decisions on participation in moderate- or vigorous-intensity exercise be based on the current level of PA and whether or not signs and symptoms of disease are present. This approach is presented in Figure 2.2 and begins with determining whether the client regularly participates in *exercise*, defined as planned, structured PA at least 30 minutes at moderate intensity for at least $3\ d \cdot wk^{-1}$ for at least the past 3 months. Regardless of the preparticipation health screening outcome, it is important to point out that periodic medical examination is imperative, as stated in *ACSM's GETP11*: "Preparticipation health screening before initiating an exercise program should be distinguished from a periodic medical examination, which should be encouraged as part of routine health maintenance."

When planning an exercise program or a fitness assessment, the first decision to be made is to determine whether a client should be advised to have medical clearance before participation in moderate- or vigorous-intensity activities, and this decision should be guided by the Preparticipation Logic Model (Figure 2.2). Alternatively and for simplification, the exercise professional may also use the exercise preparticipation health screening questionnaire for exercise professionals (Figure 2.3). For each client, the exercise professional should use the following directions as a guide (4):

- For clients who are currently *active*:
  - If asymptomatic without known CV, metabolic, or renal diseases, one may continue the exercise program and may progress gradually using published ACSM guidelines (3).

TABLE 2.1 • Major Signs or Symptoms Suggestive of Cardiovascular, Metabolic, or Renal Disease

Pain: discomfort (or other anginal equivalent) in the chest, neck, jaw, arms, or other areas that may result from myocardial ischemia; or other recent-onset pain of unknown origin
Shortness of breath at rest or with mild exertion
Dizziness or syncope
Orthopnea or paroxysmal nocturnal dyspnea
Ankle edema
Palpitations or tachycardia
Intermittent claudication
Known heart murmur
Unusual fatigue or shortness of breath with usual activities

For more explanation of these signs and symptoms, see *GETP11* Table 2.1.

Exercise Preparticipation Health Screening Questionnaire for Exercise Professionals

Assess your client's health needs by marking all _true_ statements.

Step 1

SIGNS AND SYMPTOMS
Does your client experience:
____ chest discomfort with exertion
____ unreasonable breathlessness
____ dizziness, fainting, blackouts
____ ankle swelling
____ unpleasant awareness of a forceful, rapid, or irregular heart rate
____ burning or cramping sensations in your lower legs when walking short distance
____ known heart murmur

If you **did** mark any of these statements under the symptoms, **STOP**, your client should seek medical clearance before engaging in or resuming exercise. Your client may need to use a facility with a **medically qualified staff**.

If you **did not** mark any symptoms, continue to Steps 2 and 3.

Step 2

CURRENT ACTIVITY
Has your client performed planned, structured physical activity for at least 30 minutes at moderate intensity on at least 3 days per week for at least the last 3 months?

Yes ☐ No ☐

Continue to Step 3.

Step 3

MEDICAL CONDITIONS
Has your client had or do they currently have:
____ a heart attack
____ heart surgery, cardiac catheterization, or coronary angioplasty
____ pacemaker/implantable cardiac defibrillator/rhythm disturbance
____ heart valve disease
____ heart failure
____ heart transplantation
____ congenital heart disease
____ diabetes
____ renal disease

Evaluating Steps 2 and 3:

- If you **did not mark any of the statements in Step 3**, medical clearance is not necessary.
- If you marked Step 2 "**yes**" and **marked any of the statements in Step 3**, your client may continue to exercise at light to moderate intensity without medical clearance. However, medical clearance is recommended before engaging in vigorous exercise.
- If you marked Step 2 "**no**" and **marked any of the statements in Step 3**, medical clearance is recommended. Your client may need to use a facility with a **medically qualified staff**.

Figure 2.3 Exercise preparticipation health screening questionnaire for exercise professionals.

- If asymptomatic with known CV, metabolic, or renal diseases, one may continue the exercise program as long as one remains symptom free and as long as medical clearance was given within the past 12 months.
- If symptomatic with or without known CV, metabolic, or renal diseases, one should discontinue the exercise program and seek medical clearance.
- For clients who are currently _inactive_:
  - If asymptomatic without known CV, metabolic, or renal diseases, one may engage in a light- to moderate-intensity exercise program and may progress gradually using published ACSM guidelines (3).
  - If asymptomatic with known CV, metabolic, or renal diseases, one should discontinue the exercise program and seek medical clearance.
  - If symptomatic with or without known CV, metabolic, or renal diseases, one should discontinue the exercise program and seek medical clearance.

It is critical to point out that the exercise preparticipation health screening recommendations are not a replacement for sound clinical judgment. Exercise professionals should always use prudent judgment when deciding whether a client needs medical clearance before the initiation of exercise program or a fitness assessment. If unsure, select the conservative option and the required medical clearance. Health care providers can provide useful personalized advice on how to reduce risk of injuries. For people who wish to seek the advice of a health care provider, it is particularly appropriate to do so when contemplating vigorous-intensity activity, because the risks of this activity are higher than the risks of moderate-intensity activity, especially in those who are not accustomed to this level of intensity and among those with advanced age (5,6).

Physical Activity Readiness Questionnaire for Everyone

As noted earlier, the PAR-Q+ (Figure 2.4) may be used as an alternative self-guided screener or as a supplemental tool for exercise professionals in addition to ACSM preparticipation screening algorithm. As stated in *GETP11*, "the cognitive ability required to fully answer the PAR-Q+, some individuals

2021 PAR-Q+

The Physical Activity Readiness Questionnaire for Everyone

The health benefits of regular physical activity are clear; more people should engage in physical activity every day of the week. Participating in physical activity is very safe for MOST people. This questionnaire will tell you whether it is necessary for you to seek further advice from your doctor OR a qualified exercise professional before becoming more physically active.

GENERAL HEALTH QUESTIONS

Please read the 7 questions below carefully and answer each one honestly: check YES or NO.	YES	NO
1) Has your doctor ever said that you have a heart condition ☐ **OR** high blood pressure ☐ ?	☐	☐
2) Do you feel pain in your chest at rest, during your daily activities of living, **OR** when you do physical activity?	☐	☐
3) Do you lose balance because of dizziness **OR** have you lost consciousness in the last 12 months? Please answer **NO** if your dizziness was associated with over-breathing (including during vigorous exercise).	☐	☐
4) Have you ever been diagnosed with another chronic medical condition (other than heart disease or high blood pressure)? **PLEASE LIST CONDITION(S) HERE:** _____	☐	☐
5) Are you currently taking prescribed medications for a chronic medical condition? **PLEASE LIST CONDITION(S) AND MEDICATIONS HERE:** _____	☐	☐
6) Do you currently have (or have had within the past 12 months) a bone, joint, or soft tissue (muscle, ligament, or tendon) problem that could be made worse by becoming more physically active? Please answer **NO** if you had a problem in the past, but it **does not limit your current ability** to be physically active. **PLEASE LIST CONDITION(S) HERE:** _____	☐	☐
7) Has your doctor ever said that you should only do medically supervised physical activity?	☐	☐

☑ **If you answered NO to all of the questions above, you are cleared for physical activity.**
Please sign the PARTICIPANT DECLARATION. You do not need to complete Pages 2 and 3.

▶ Start becoming much more physically active – start slowly and build up gradually.

▶ Follow Global Physical Activity Guidelines for your age (https://apps.who.int/iris/handle/10665/44399).

▶ You may take part in a health and fitness appraisal.

▶ If you are over the age of 45 yr and NOT accustomed to regular vigorous to maximal effort exercise, consult a qualified exercise professional before engaging in this intensity of exercise.

▶ If you have any further questions, contact a qualified exercise professional.

PARTICIPANT DECLARATION
If you are less than the legal age required for consent or require the assent of a care provider, your parent, guardian or care provider must also sign this form.

I, the undersigned, have read, understood to my full satisfaction and completed this questionnaire. I acknowledge that this physical activity clearance is valid for a maximum of 12 months from the date it is completed and becomes invalid if my condition changes. I also acknowledge that the community/fitness center may retain a copy of this form for its records. In these instances, it will maintain the confidentiality of the same, complying with applicable law.

NAME _____ DATE _____

SIGNATURE _____ WITNESS _____

SIGNATURE OF PARENT/GUARDIAN/CARE PROVIDER _____

⬤ **If you answered YES to one or more of the questions above, COMPLETE PAGES 2 AND 3.**

⚠ **Delay becoming more active if:**

✎ You have a temporary illness such as a cold or fever; it is best to wait until you feel better.

✎ You are pregnant - talk to your health care practitioner, your physician, a qualified exercise professional, and/or complete the ePARmed-X+ at www.eparmedx.com before becoming more physically active.

✎ Your health changes - answer the questions on Pages 2 and 3 of this document and/or talk to your doctor or a qualified exercise professional before continuing with any physical activity program.

Figure 2.4 The Physical Activity Readiness Questionnaire + (PAR-Q+).

2021 PAR-Q+

FOLLOW-UP QUESTIONS ABOUT YOUR MEDICAL CONDITION(S)

1.   Do you have Arthritis, Osteoporosis, or Back Problems?

If the above condition(s) is/are present, answer questions 1a-1c   If **NO** ☐ go to question 2

1a.	Do you have difficulty controlling your condition with medications or other physician-prescribed therapies? (Answer **NO** if you are not currently taking medications or other treatments)	YES ☐ NO ☐
1b.	Do you have joint problems causing pain, a recent fracture or fracture caused by osteoporosis or cancer, displaced vertebra (e.g., spondylolisthesis), and/or spondylolysis/pars defect (a crack in the bony ring on the back of the spinal column)?	YES ☐ NO ☐
1c.	Have you had steroid injections or taken steroid tablets regularly for more than 3 months?	YES ☐ NO ☐

2.   Do you currently have Cancer of any kind?

If the above condition(s) is/are present, answer questions 2a-2b   If **NO** ☐ go to question 3

2a.	Does your cancer diagnosis include any of the following types: lung/bronchogenic, multiple myeloma (cancer of plasma cells), head, and/or neck?	YES ☐ NO ☐
2b.	Are you currently receiving cancer therapy (such as chemotheraphy or radiotherapy)?	YES ☐ NO ☐

3.   Do you have a Heart or Cardiovascular Condition? This includes Coronary Artery Disease, Heart Failure, Diagnosed Abnormality of Heart Rhythm

If the above condition(s) is/are present, answer questions 3a-3d   If **NO** ☐ go to question 4

3a.	Do you have difficulty controlling your condition with medications or other physician-prescribed therapies? (Answer **NO** if you are not currently taking medications or other treatments)	YES ☐ NO ☐
3b.	Do you have an irregular heart beat that requires medical management? (e.g., atrial fibrillation, premature ventricular contraction)	YES ☐ NO ☐
3c.	Do you have chronic heart failure?	YES ☐ NO ☐
3d.	Do you have diagnosed coronary artery (cardiovascular) disease and have not participated in regular physical activity in the last 2 months?	YES ☐ NO ☐

4.   Do you currently have High Blood Pressure?

If the above condition(s) is/are present, answer questions 4a-4b   If **NO** ☐ go to question 5

4a.	Do you have difficulty controlling your condition with medications or other physician-prescribed therapies? (Answer **NO** if you are not currently taking medications or other treatments)	YES ☐ NO ☐
4b.	Do you have a resting blood pressure equal to or greater than 160/90 mmHg with or without medication? (Answer **YES** if you do not know your resting blood pressure)	YES ☐ NO ☐

5.   Do you have any Metabolic Conditions? This includes Type 1 Diabetes, Type 2 Diabetes, Pre-Diabetes

If the above condition(s) is/are present, answer questions 5a-5e   If **NO** ☐ go to question 6

5a.	Do you often have difficulty controlling your blood sugar levels with foods, medications, or other physician-prescribed therapies?	YES ☐ NO ☐
5b.	Do you often suffer from signs and symptoms of low blood sugar (hypoglycemia) following exercise and/or during activities of daily living? Signs of hypoglycemia may include shakiness, nervousness, unusual irritability, abnormal sweating, dizziness or light-headedness, mental confusion, difficulty speaking, weakness, or sleepiness.	YES ☐ NO ☐
5c.	Do you have any signs or symptoms of diabetes complications such as heart or vascular disease and/or complications affecting your eyes, kidneys, **OR** the sensation in your toes and feet?	YES ☐ NO ☐
5d.	Do you have other metabolic conditions (such as current pregnancy-related diabetes, chronic kidney disease, or liver problems)?	YES ☐ NO ☐
5e.	Are you planning to engage in what for you is unusually high (or vigorous) intensity exercise in the near future?	YES ☐ NO ☐

Figure 2.4 *(continued)*

2021 PAR-Q+

6. **Do you have any Mental Health Problems or Learning Difficulties?** This includes Alzheimer's, Dementia, Depression, Anxiety Disorder, Eating Disorder, Psychotic Disorder, Intellectual Disability, Down Syndrome

If the above condition(s) is/are present, answer questions 6a-6b   If **NO** ☐ go to question 7

6a.	Do you have difficulty controlling your condition with medications or other physician-prescribed therapies? (Answer **NO** if you are not currently taking medications or other treatments)	YES ☐ NO ☐
6b.	Do you have Down Syndrome **AND** back problems affecting nerves or muscles?	YES ☐ NO ☐

7. **Do you have a Respiratory Disease?** This includes Chronic Obstructive Pulmonary Disease, Asthma, Pulmonary High Blood Pressure

If the above condition(s) is/are present, answer questions 7a-7d   If **NO** ☐ go to question 8

7a.	Do you have difficulty controlling your condition with medications or other physician-prescribed therapies? (Answer **NO** if you are not currently taking medications or other treatments)	YES ☐ NO ☐
7b.	Has your doctor ever said your blood oxygen level is low at rest or during exercise and/or that you require supplemental oxygen therapy?	YES ☐ NO ☐
7c.	If asthmatic, do you currently have symptoms of chest tightness, wheezing, laboured breathing, consistent cough (more than 2 days/week), or have you used your rescue medication more than twice in the last week?	YES ☐ NO ☐
7d.	Has your doctor ever said you have high blood pressure in the blood vessels of your lungs?	YES ☐ NO ☐

8. **Do you have a Spinal Cord Injury?** This includes Tetraplegia and Paraplegia

If the above condition(s) is/are present, answer questions 8a-8c   If **NO** ☐ go to question 9

8a.	Do you have difficulty controlling your condition with medications or other physician-prescribed therapies? (Answer **NO** if you are not currently taking medications or other treatments)	YES ☐ NO ☐
8b.	Do you commonly exhibit low resting blood pressure significant enough to cause dizziness, light-headedness, and/or fainting?	YES ☐ NO ☐
8c.	Has your physician indicated that you exhibit sudden bouts of high blood pressure (known as Autonomic Dysreflexia)?	YES ☐ NO ☐

9. **Have you had a Stroke?** This includes Transient Ischemic Attack (TIA) or Cerebrovascular Event

If the above condition(s) is/are present, answer questions 9a-9c   If **NO** ☐ go to question 10

9a.	Do you have difficulty controlling your condition with medications or other physician-prescribed therapies? (Answer **NO** if you are not currently taking medications or other treatments)	YES ☐ NO ☐
9b.	Do you have any impairment in walking or mobility?	YES ☐ NO ☐
9c.	Have you experienced a stroke or impairment in nerves or muscles in the past 6 months?	YES ☐ NO ☐

10. **Do you have any other medical condition not listed above or do you have two or more medical conditions?**

If you have other medical conditions, answer questions 10a-10c   If **NO** ☐ read the Page 4 recommendations

10a.	Have you experienced a blackout, fainted, or lost consciousness as a result of a head injury within the last 12 months **OR** have you had a diagnosed concussion within the last 12 months?	YES ☐ NO ☐
10b.	Do you have a medical condition that is not listed (such as epilepsy, neurological conditions, kidney problems)?	YES ☐ NO ☐
10c.	Do you currently live with two or more medical conditions?	YES ☐ NO ☐

PLEASE LIST YOUR MEDICAL CONDITION(S) AND ANY RELATED MEDICATIONS HERE: _____

_____

GO to Page 4 for recommendations about your current medical condition(s) and sign the PARTICIPANT DECLARATION.

Figure 2.4 *(continued)*

2021 PAR-Q+

☑ **If you answered NO to all of the FOLLOW-UP questions (pgs. 2-3) about your medical condition, you are ready to become more physically active - sign the PARTICIPANT DECLARATION below:**

▶ It is advised that you consult a qualified exercise professional to help you develop a safe and effective physical activity plan to meet your health needs.

▶ You are encouraged to start slowly and build up gradually - 20 to 60 minutes of low to moderate intensity exercise, 3-5 days per week including aerobic and muscle strengthening exercises.

▶ As you progress, you should aim to accumulate 150 minutes or more of moderate intensity physical activity per week.

▶ If you are over the age of 45 yr and **NOT** accustomed to regular vigorous to maximal effort exercise, consult a qualified exercise professional before engaging in this intensity of exercise.

◉ **If you answered YES to one or more of the follow-up questions about your medical condition:**

You should seek further information before becoming more physically active or engaging in a fitness appraisal. You should complete the specially designed online screening and exercise recommendations program - the **ePARmed-X+ at www.eparmedx.com** and/or visit a qualified exercise professional to work through the ePARmed-X+ and for further information.

⚠ **Delay becoming more active if:**

You have a temporary illness such as a cold or fever; it is best to wait until you feel better.

You are pregnant - talk to your health care practitioner, your physician, a qualified exercise professional, and/or complete the ePARmed-X+ **at www.eparmedx.com** before becoming more physically active.

Your health changes - talk to your doctor or qualified exercise professional before continuing with any physical activity program.

● You are encouraged to photocopy the PAR-Q+. You must use the entire questionnaire and NO changes are permitted.
● The authors, the PAR-Q+ Collaboration, partner organizations, and their agents assume no liability for persons who undertake physical activity and/or make use of the PAR-Q+ or ePARmed-X+. If in doubt after completing the questionnaire, consult your doctor prior to physical activity.

PARTICIPANT DECLARATION

● All persons who have completed the PAR-Q+ please read and sign the declaration below.

● If you are less than the legal age required for consent or require the assent of a care provider, your parent, guardian or care provider must also sign this form.

I, the undersigned, have read, understood to my full satisfaction and completed this questionnaire. I acknowledge that this physical activity clearance is valid for a maximum of 12 months from the date it is completed and becomes invalid if my condition changes. I also acknowledge that the community/fitness center may retain a copy of this form for records. In these instances, it will maintain the confidentiality of the same, complying with applicable law.

NAME _____ DATE _____

SIGNATURE _____ WITNESS _____

SIGNATURE OF PARENT/GUARDIAN/CARE PROVIDER _____

———— For more information, please contact ————
www.eparmedx.com
Email: eparmedx@gmail.com

Citation for PAR-Q+
Warburton DER, Jamnik VK, Bredin SSD, and Gledhill N on behalf of the PAR-Q+ Collaboration. The Physical Activity Readiness Questionnaire for Everyone (PAR-Q+) and Electronic Physical Activity Readiness Medical Examination (ePARmed-X+). Health & Fitness Journal of Canada 4(2):3-23, 2011.

Key References
1. Jamnik VK, Warburton DER, Makarski J, McKenzie DC, Shephard RJ, Stone J, and Gledhill N. Enhancing the effectiveness of clearance for physical activity participation; background and overall process. APNM 36(S1):S3-S13, 2011.
2. Warburton DER, Gledhill N, Jamnik VK, Bredin SSD, McKenzie DC, Stone J, Charlesworth S, and Shephard RJ. Evidence-based risk assessment and recommendations for physical activity clearance; Consensus Document. APNM 36(S1):S266-s298, 2011.
3. Chisholm DM, Collis ML, Kulak LL, Davenport W, and Gruber N. Physical activity readiness. British Columbia Medical Journal. 1975;17:375-378.
4. Thomas S, Reading J, and Shephard RJ. Revision of the Physical Activity Readiness Questionnaire (PAR-Q). Canadian Journal of Sport Science 1992;17:4 338-345.

The PAR-Q+ was created using the evidence-based AGREE process (1) by the PAR-Q+ Collaboration chaired by Dr. Darren E. R. Warburton with Dr. Norman Gledhill, Dr. Veronica Jamnik, and Dr. Donald C. McKenzie (2). Production of this document has been made possible through financial contributions from the Public Health Agency of Canada and the BC Ministry of Health Services. The views expressed herein do not necessarily represent the views of the Public Health Agency of Canada or the BC Ministry of Health Services.

Figure 2.4 (*continued*)

may require assistance completing the assessment." Exercise professionals should facilitate a follow-up process with the client to ensure that the document is completed fully and to answer any follow-up questions.

Exercise Testing

Although ACSM preparticipation algorithm provides guidance for exercise preparticipation screening, this procedure should not be used as a sole screening tool prior to conducting exercise testing and should be used in conjunction with other tools, such as a health history questionnaire (HHQ) (3). Regardless of the need for medical clearance, there still may be times when an exercise test is conducted as part of a fitness assessment. If an exercise test is elected, ACSM supports that these tests can be supervised by an appropriately trained allied health professional or clinical exercise physiologist, because

Box 2.2	Contraindications to Symptom-Limited Maximal Exercise Testing

Absolute

- A recent significant change in the resting electrocardiogram suggesting significant ischemia, recent myocardial infarction (within 2 d), or other acute cardiac event
- Unstable angina
- Uncontrolled cardiac dysrhythmias causing symptoms or hemodynamic compromise
- Symptomatic severe aortic stenosis
- Uncontrolled symptomatic heart failure
- Acute pulmonary embolus or pulmonary infarction
- Acute myocarditis or pericarditis
- Suspected or known dissecting aneurysm
- Acute systemic infection, accompanied by fever, body aches, or swollen lymph glands

Relative[a]

- Left main coronary stenosis
- Moderate stenotic valvular heart disease
- Electrolyte abnormalities (*e.g.*, hypokalemia, hypomagnesemia)
- Severe arterial hypertension (*i.e.*, SBP of >200 mm Hg and/or a DBP of >110 mm Hg) at rest
- Tachydysrhythmia or bradydysrhythmia
- Hypertrophic cardiomyopathy and other forms of outflow tract obstruction
- Neuromotor, musculoskeletal, or rheumatoid disorders that are exacerbated by exercise
- High-degree atrioventricular block
- Ventricular aneurysm
- Uncontrolled metabolic disease (*e.g.*, diabetes, thyrotoxicosis, myxedema)
- Chronic infectious disease (*e.g.*, human immunodeficiency virus)
- Mental or physical impairment leading to inability to exercise adequately

[a]Relative contraindications can be superseded if benefits outweigh the risks of exercise. In some instances, these individuals can be exercised with caution and/or using low-level end points, especially if they are asymptomatic at rest.
Modified from Fletcher GF, Ades PA, Kligfield P, et al. Exercise standards for testing and training: a scientific statement from the American Heart Association. *Circulation*. 2013;128(8):873–934 (40).

there are no differences in morbidity and mortality rates when conducted by appropriately trained staff compared to physician-supervised tests (7). It is important to understand that this process is only a recommended guide for action as no set of exercise guidelines covers all the different situations related to preparticipation screening; therefore, it is always necessary to be cognizant of local policies and procedures. Exercise professionals should also be aware of contraindications to exercise and exercise testing. It is critically important to recognize that a client may have medical conditions for which exercise should not be performed until the condition is resolved. These are conditions for which the immediate risks of exercise outweigh any potential benefit that could be derived from the exercise. These are called contraindications to symptom-limited maximal exercise testing and are listed in Box 2.2. Clients identified with these factors should seek medical attention for the condition prior to performing a fitness assessment.

Health History Questionnaire

Most of the pertinent health risks and medical information about a client can be obtained from an HHQ. A well-designed HHQ should note the individual's current activity habits; identify any serious medical conditions (contraindications to exercise); document any known CVD, pulmonary disease, or renal disease, or the presence of diabetes; and determine CVD risk factors. The HHQ can be tailored to fit the specific information required of the type of fitness assessment being performed. For example, little health risk and medical information is needed if the client is only performing a body composition assessment. However, clients interested in performing assessments requiring maximal exercise should complete a comprehensive HHQ. In general, the HHQ should assess a client's:

- CVD risk factors.
- past history and present status of any signs and symptoms suggestive of CVD.
- history of chronic diseases and illnesses.
- history of surgeries and hospitalizations.

- history of any MSI and joint injury.
- past and present health behaviors/habits (PA, dietary patterns, and weight loss).
- current use of any prescribed or over-the-counter (OTC) medications.

An example of a comprehensive health history form is shown in Figure 2.5.

Cardiovascular Disease Risk Factors

The CVD risk factor thresholds of ACSM are listed in Table 2.2. ACSM uses risk factor criteria established by other professional organizations, such as the American Association of Clinical Endocrinologists and the American College of Endocrinology (8). However, slightly different risk factor criteria may be found in some other sources.

TODAY'S DATE _____

NAME _____ AGE _____ DATE OF BIRTH _____

ADDRESS _____
                    Street   City   State   Zip

TELEPHONE: HOME/CELL _____/ _____ E-MAIL ADDRESS _____

OCCUPATION/EMPLOYER _____/ _____ BUSINESS PHONE _____

MARITAL STATUS: (check one) SINGLE ☐   MARRIED ☐   DIVORCED ☐   WIDOWED ☐

PERSONAL PHYSICIAN _____ PHONE # _____

ADDRESS _____

Reason for last doctor visit?_____ Date of last physical exam: _____

Have you ever had any other exercise stress test?   YES ☐   NO ☐   DATE & LOCATION OF TEST: _____

_____

Have you ever had any cardiovascular tests?   YES ☐   NO ☐   DATE & LOCATION: _____

_____

Person to contact in case of an emergency _____ Phone _____ (relationship) _____

Please provide responses (YES or NO) to the following concerning family history, your own history, and any symptoms you have had:

FAMILY HISTORY			PERSONAL HISTORY			SYMPTOMS		
Have any immediate family members had a:	YES	NO	Have you ever had:	YES	NO	Have you ever had:	YES	NO
heart attack	o	o	High blood pressure	o	o	Chest pain	o	o
heart surgery	o	o	High cholesterol	o	o	Shortness of breath	o	o
coronary stent	o	o	Diabetes	o	o	Heart palpitations	o	o
cardiac catheterization	o	o	Any heart problems	o	o	Skipped heartbeats	o	o
congenital heart defect	o	o	Disease of arteries	o	o	Heart murmur	o	o
stroke	o	o	Thyroid disease	o	o	Intermittent leg pain	o	o
Other chronic disease: _____			Lung disease	o	o	Dizziness or fainting	o	o
_____			Asthma	o	o	Fatigue — usual activities	o	o
_____			Cancer	o	o	Snoring	o	o
_____			Kidney disease	o	o	Back pain	o	o
_____			Hepatitis	o	o	Orthopedic problems	o	o
			Other: _____			Other: _____		

STAFF COMMENTS: _____

_____

_____

Have you ever had your cholesterol measured?   Yes ☐   No ☐   If yes, value _____ Where: _____

Are you taking any prescription (include birth control pills) or nonprescription medications?   Yes ☐   No ☐
For each of your current medications, provide the following information:

MEDICATION   Dosage—times/day   Time taken   Years on medication   Reason for taking

_____

_____

_____

HOSPITALIZATIONS: Please list recent hospitalizations (Women: do not list normal pregnancies)

Figure 2.5 An example of a comprehensive health history questionnaire. Source: Ball State University—Clinical Exercise Physiology Program.

TABLE 2.2 • Cardiovascular Disease (CVD) Risk Factors and Defining Criteria

Positive Risk Factors[a]	Defining Criteria
Age	Men ≥ 45 yr; women ≥ 55 yr (35)
Family history	Myocardial infarction, coronary revascularization, or sudden death before 55 yr in father or other male first-degree relative or before 65 yr in mother or other female first-degree relative (36)
Cigarette smoking	Current cigarette smoker or those who quit within the previous 6 mo or exposure to environmental tobacco smoke (36,37)
Physical inactivity	Not meeting the minimum threshold of 500–1,000 MET-minutes of moderate- to vigorous-intensity physical activity, or 75–150 min · wk^{-1} of moderate- to vigorous-intensity physical activity (28)
Body mass index/waist circumference	Body mass index ≥ 30 kg · m^{-2} or waist girth > 102 cm (40 in) for men and > 88 cm (35 in) for women (38)
Blood pressure	Systolic blood pressure ≥ 130 mm Hg and/or diastolic ≥ 80 mm Hg, based on an average of ≥2 readings obtained on ≥2 occasions, or on antihypertensive medication (39)
Lipids	Low-density lipoprotein cholesterol (LDL-C) ≥130 mg · dL^{-1} (3.37 mmol · L^{-1}) or high-density lipoprotein cholesterol (HDL-C) <40 mg · dL^{-1} (1.04 mmol · L^{-1}) in men and <50 mg · dL^{-1} (1.30 mmol · L^{-1}) in women or non-HDL-C ≥160 (4.14 mmol · L^{-1}) or on lipid-lowering medication. If total serum cholesterol is all that is available, use ≥200 mg · dL^{-1} (5.18 mmol · L^{-1}) (8)
Blood glucose	Fasting plasma glucose ≥ 100 mg · dL^{-1} (5.5 mmol · L^{-1}); or 2 h plasma glucose values in oral glucose tolerance test (OGTT) ≥ 140 mg · dL^{-1} (7.77 mmol · L^{-1}); or hemoglobin A1C ≥ 5.7% (20)
Negative Risk Factors	**Defining Criteria**
HDL-C[b]	≥60 mg · dL^{-1} (1.55 mmol · L^{-1}) (8)

[a]If the presence or absence of a CVD risk factor is not disclosed or is not available, that CVD risk factor should be counted as a risk factor.

[b]High HDL-C is considered a negative risk factor. For individuals having high HDL ≥ 60 mg · dL^{-1} (1.55 mmol · L^{-1}), one positive risk factor is subtracted from the sum of positive risk factors.

It is important to follow the specific criteria for determining the presence or absence of each CVD risk factor. For example, note that age thresholds differ between the age risk factor and the family history risk factor. In addition, for the BP risk factor, repeat assessments are necessary to confirm the measurement. Furthermore and for BP and lipids risk factors, those whose conditions are controlled by medications are still considered to have the respective risk factors. The risk factor analysis is important and may be used for the development of exercise prescriptions, the need for lifestyle modifications, and patient education about CVD risk reduction.

Note that there are eight positive risk factors and one negative risk factor identified by ACSM. If a client has high high-density lipoprotein cholesterol (HDL-C), then one positive risk factor is subtracted from the sum of the positive risk factors to determine the total number of risk factors. Risk factor identification should be used both for client education and for developing appropriate exercise prescriptions.

OTHER HEALTH ISSUES TO CONSIDER

ACSM screening guidelines focus on current exercise level and signs and symptoms suggestive of disease. The American Heart Association screening recommendations are focused mostly on CVD risk issues (9). Neither of these organizations emphasize a medical history of musculoskeletal problems; however, if this is present, then a similar referral to a health care provider should be made before any fitness assessment that could impact the musculoskeletal condition.

Understanding Medication Usage

A list of all medications that a client is presently using should be obtained during the preassessment screening. It is beyond the level of expertise for a nonclinical exercise professional to have a complete understanding of all medications. However, the exercise professional should minimally know if a client is taking any medications and whether the medication may alter the client's response to acute or chronic exercise. There are many sources to review medications, their side effects, and how they impact the exercise response. Some sources are quite detailed and are beyond the scope of information needed by the exercise professional. The U.S. National Library of Medicine and the National Institutes of Health provide a straightforward Web site that allows for a search of a specific medication and yields information regarding usage, side effects, and precautions (10). In addition, *ACSM's GETP11* provides information on medications in appendix A (3).

The exercise professional should not instruct a client to stop taking or change the timing of his or her medication before any fitness assessment. Only the client's physician should make such decisions.

RATIONALE FOR RISK ASSESSMENT

A client who is an active participant in his or her health care will likely have many risk factors measured and monitored through regular medical checkups. These individuals can provide most of the necessary risk assessment information via self-report in an HHQ. However, many clients may not regularly see a physician or may not have had these measurements taken for over a year. Thus, an important service for personnel who provide fitness assessments is to also provide measurements of common risk factors and screenings for other chronic diseases. In addition, these measures may stimulate a client to pay more attention to specific personal health when risk factors are detected, motivating them to make positive health-related changes. In some cases, results may even identify individuals who need to seek medical follow-up.

CARDIOVASCULAR HEMODYNAMICS

The CV system acts as the pump for the blood to the body, with the heart serving as the pulsatile pump. The term for the overall function of the CV system is the *cardiovascular hemodynamics* or *cardiac function*. BP and HR make up some of the variables responsible for the CV hemodynamics. The multiplication of systolic BP (SBP) by HR is known as the *rate pressure product* (RPP) or *double product* (DP), and it is a useful tool for exercise prescription as a measure of myocardial oxygen demand.

Resting Blood Pressure

BP is the force of blood exerted against the walls of the arteries and veins created by the heart as it pumps blood to every part of the body. For a health risk assessment, arterial BP is measured and expressed in units of millimeters of mercury (mm Hg), and there are two phases assessed, systolic pressure and diastolic pressure. SBP is the maximum pressure in the arteries during the contraction (systole) phase of the heart cycle. The diastolic BP (DBP) is the minimum pressure in the arteries during the relaxation (diastole) phase of the heart cycle. BP measurements are used in determining total number of risk factors present and how to proceed with an exercise prescription and health education.

Measurement

The direct measure of BP requires an invasive procedure that can only be performed by a trained clinical professional and involves the placement of a catheter in an artery followed by the insertion of a pressure transducer into the catheter (11). Therefore, fitness assessments use an indirect method of measuring BP termed *auscultation*, which involves listening to internal sounds of the body using a stethoscope. For BP assessment, a stethoscope is placed over an artery to listen for the Korotkoff sounds on the arterial walls (see Box 2.3). The Korotkoff sounds heard through the stethoscope during the BP measurement come from the turbulence of blood in the artery, which is caused by blood moving from an area of higher pressure to an area of lower pressure. A cuff is applied to the upper arm and is inflated with air by pumping a hand bulb. The ensuing air pressure inside the BP cuff occludes the blood flow within the brachial artery, and as long as the pressure in the cuff is higher than the SBP, the artery remains occluded or collapsed, and no sound is heard through the applied stethoscope. When the air pressure is slowly released from the cuff, the pressure inside the cuff will eventually equal the driving

> ## Box 2.3   Korotkoff Sounds
>
> - Phase 1. The first, initial sound or the onset of sound. Sounds like clear, repetitive tapping. The sound may be faint at first and gradually increase in intensity or volume to phase 2.
> - Phase 2. Sounds like a soft tapping or murmur. The sounds are often longer than the phase 1 sounds. These sounds have also been described as having a swishing component. The phase 2 sounds are typically 10 to 15 mm Hg after the onset of sound (phase 1).
> - Phase 3. Sounds like a loud tapping sound; high in both pitch and intensity. These sounds are crisper and louder than the phase 2 sounds.
> - Phase 4. Sounds like a muffling of the sound. The sounds become less distinct and less audible. Another way of describing this sound is as soft or blowing.
> - Phase 5. Sounds like the complete disappearance of sound. The true disappearance of sound usually occurs within 8 to 10 mm Hg of the muffling of sound (phase 4).

pressure of the blood in the artery, and the first sound will be heard in the stethoscope. This sound corresponds to the measure of SBP. As the pressure in the cuff continues to drop, it will eventually get to a point where the cuff is no longer occluding the artery, and all sounds will disappear as blood flow returns to normal. The pressure reading at the last sound heard is the DBP.

Measurement Equipment BP measurement using the auscultatory method requires a stethoscope, a manometer or sphygmomanometer (a device to measure pressure), and a cuff with an inflatable bladder that is wrapped around the limb (typically the arm). The two common types of manometers used for BP measurement are mercury and aneroid, as shown in Figure 2.6. Mercury, the standard for pressure measurements, is housed in a small reservoir (~300 mm) located at the base of a vertical glass column. However, because mercury is a toxic chemical, aneroid sphygmomanometers are becoming more common in the workplace. Indeed, many facilities have instituted a ban on all devices containing mercury. Further, regulations for disposal of mercury must be followed and vary by state. Knowledge of state and facility regulations regarding mercury use and disposal is imperative and can be researched through the U.S. Environmental Protection Agency (12).

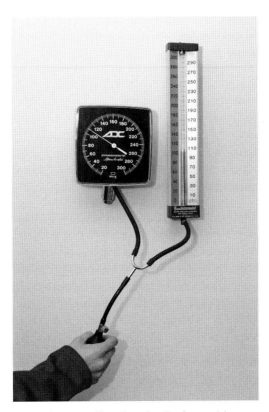

Figure 2.6 A Y tube is used to perform a calibration check of aneroid manometers. Source: Photograph by Ball State University.

Box 2.4   Procedures for Assessment of Resting Blood Pressure

1. Patients should be seated quietly for at least 5 min in a chair with back support (rather than on an examination table) with their feet on the floor and their arms supported at heart level. Patients should refrain from smoking cigarettes or ingesting caffeine for at least 30 min preceding the measurement.
2. Measuring supine and standing values may be indicated under special circumstances.
3. Wrap cuff firmly around upper arm at heart level; align cuff with brachial artery.
4. The appropriate cuff size must be used to ensure accurate measurement. The bladder within the cuff should encircle at least 80% of the upper arm. Many adults require a large adult cuff.
5. Place stethoscope chest piece below the antecubital space over the brachial artery. Bell and diaphragm side of chest piece appear equally effective in assessing BP (41).
6. Quickly inflate cuff pressure to 20 mm Hg above the first Korotkoff sound.
7. Slowly release pressure at a rate equal to 2 to 3 mm Hg $\cdot$ s^{-1}.
8. SBP is the point at which the first of two or more Korotkoff sounds is heard (phase 1), and DBP is the point before the disappearance of Korotkoff sounds (phase 5).
9. At least two measurements should be made (minimum of 1 min apart), and the average should be taken.
10. BP should be measured in both arms during the first examination. Higher pressure should be used when there is consistent interarm difference.
11. Provide to patients, verbally and in writing, their specific BP numbers and BP goals.

Data from Whelton PK, Carey RM, Aronow WS, et al. 2017 ACC/AHA/AAPA/ABC/ACPM/AGS/APhA/ASH/ASPC/NMA/PCNA guideline for the prevention, detection, evaluation, and management of high blood pressure in adults: a report of the American College of Cardiology/American Heart Association Task Force on Clinical Practice Guidelines. *J Am Coll Cardiol*. 2018;71(19):e127–e248. For additional, more detailed recommendations, see reference [11].

Aneroid sphygmomanometers measure the pressure in the cuff by the movement of a spring-loaded needle that moves on a dial-type scale. Facilities should have at least three different BP cuff sizes available: small, medium, and large. There are index lines on most sphygmomanometer cuffs to help determine the correct cuff for a client's arm circumference. Typically, the appropriate BP bladder (the inflatable rubber sac within the cuff) should encircle at least 80% of the arm's circumference without overlapping. In general, a bladder within the cuff that is too small will result in an overestimation of BP, and a cuff that is too long will result in an underestimation of BP.

Equipment used in the measurement of BP is widely available commercially but varies greatly in quality. Sphygmomanometer units and stethoscopes can be purchased in most pharmacies, various health and fitness commercial catalogs, and medical supply stores. A high-quality stethoscope is worth the investment to help in hearing clear Korotkoff sounds.

Automated Systems Electronic BP machines have been available for many years, and industrial models are increasingly being used in both hospitals and doctors' offices. Commercial models have also become relatively inexpensive for individuals who wish to self-monitor BP at home (13). Most of these systems use the oscillatory method for measuring BP, in which the cuff is filled with fluid instead of air. SBP is detected when oscillations begin during the deflation of the pressure, with DBP being recorded at the point of maximal oscillations. Although these devices have been shown to provide reasonably accurate BP measurements, they are difficult to calibrate over time.

Assessment Technique For accurate resting BP readings, it is important that the client be made as comfortable as possible. As with many other physiologic and psychological measures taken, there exists what is called the "white coat syndrome" in the measurement of BP. This *white coat syndrome* refers to an elevation of BP because of the effect of being in a doctor's office or in a clinical setting (*i.e.*, clinician wearing a white lab coat). The recommended standardized procedures for assessing resting BP are listed in Box 2.4.

When an individual is beginning to learn the skill of BP measurement, it is helpful to work with an experienced technician who can listen with the trainee by using a dual head (two sets of listening tubes/earpieces) or teaching stethoscope, as shown in Figure 2.7. Some helpful technique tips are as follows:

- Ideally, the client cuff should be applied to bare skin. However, thin clothing on the arm where the stethoscope is placed should not interfere with the measurement, except for the slightly lower intensity of the sound. If clothing is between the arm and the stethoscope and it is difficult to hear the Korotkoff sounds, then the procedure should be repeated with the arm bared. (Note: As a general rule, avoid rolling up the client's sleeve if the clothing becomes too tight on the upper arm because this can influence the BP because of partial occlusion of the blood vessel.)

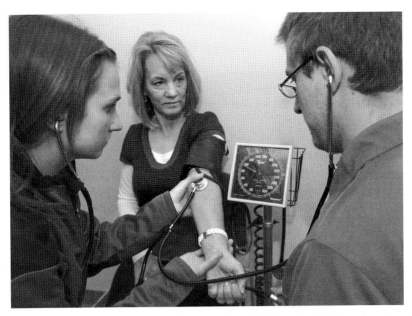

Figure 2.7 Use of a double-headed stethoscope for training technicians learning to measure blood pressure. Source: Photograph by Ball State University.

- Locate the client's brachial artery (position with the palm up and arm rotated outward on the thumb side with the arm hyperextended). This artery, and thus pulse, is just medial to the biceps tendon. Mark the artery with an appropriate marker (watercolor) for the stethoscope bell placement, especially if the BP will be assessed again during exercise.
- Firmly place the bell of the stethoscope over the brachial artery. Avoid placing the bell of the stethoscope under the lip of the BP cuff.
- The stethoscope earpieces should be facing forward, toward the nose, in the same direction as the ear canal. (Note: If a stethoscope is being shared, the earpieces should be cleaned between users.)
- Position the manometer (either mercury or aneroid) so that the manometer is clearly visible and at eye level to avoid any parallax (distortion from looking up or down) error.
- After identifying the SBP, the pressure can be lowered $\approx$20 mm Hg rapidly and then slowed to the standard deflation rate of 2 to 3 mm Hg $\cdot$ s^{-1}. More rapid deflation leads to errors in the identification of DBP.
- Record both the fourth and fifth phase sounds if clearly heard. Always record only even numbers and round off upward to the nearest 2 mm Hg. Always continue to listen for any BP sounds for at least 10 mm Hg below the fifth phase.
- If needed, it is possible to increase the intensity, or loudness, of the brachial pulse sounds by either having the client raise the arm and rapidly make a tight fist and then relax the hand 5 to 10 times or hold the arm overhead for 60 seconds. Immediately inflate the cuff after either of these procedures.

Interpretation

As noted in Table 2.2, the criteria for the hypertension risk factor are an SBP of $\geq$130 mm Hg and/or a DBP of $\geq$80 mm Hg. Remember that high readings need to be confirmed by at least one other reading on a separate day. Also note that only physicians can make a diagnosis of hypertension. Exercise professionals should inform clients if their BP is elevated in the hypertensive range and recommend they follow up with their health care provider.

More detailed classifications of resting BP readings are found in Table 2.3. These classifications, which are from the "2017 Guideline for the Prevention, Detection, Evaluation, and Management of High Blood Pressure in Adults" (14), also contain recommendations for patient follow-up. Exercise professionals should be familiar with at least the recommendations contained in the executive summary of this report.

Heart Rate

HR is defined as the number of times that the heart contracts, usually expressed in a 1-minute time frame and reported as beats per minute (bpm). There are no known or accepted standards for resting HR. Resting HR has been thought of as an indicator of CV endurance as it tends to lower as one

TABLE 2.3 • Classification and Management of Blood Pressure for Adults[a]

	ACC/AHA (2017)			
BP Classification	Normal	Elevated	Stage 1 Hypertension	Stage 2 Hypertension
SBP (mm Hg)	<120	120–129	130–139	≥140
	and	and	or	or
DBP (mm Hg)	<80	<80	80–89	≥90
Treatment recommendations	Promote optimal lifestyle habits; reassess yearly	Nonpharmacologic therapy; reassess in 3–6 mo	Clinical ASCVD or estimated 10 yr CVD risk ≥ 10%? *No: nonpharmacologic treatment; reassess in 3–6 mo Yes: continue nonphar-macologic treatment and initiate BP-lower-ing medication; follow up monthly until BP is controlled	Nonpharmacologic treatment and BP-lowering medication; follow up monthly until BP is controlled

[a]Individuals are classified in any given category by meeting either of SBP or DBP thresholds.
ACC, American College of Cardiology; AHA, American Heart Association; ASCVD, atherosclerotic cardiovas-cular disease; BP, blood pressure; CVD, cardiovascular disease; DBP, diastolic blood pressure; SBP, systolic blood pressure.
Reprinted with permission, https://www.heart.org/-/media/files/health-topics/high-blood-pressure/hbprainbow-chart-english.pdf © American Heart Association, Inc.

becomes more aerobically fit. There are also no standards for exercise HR, but the HR response to a standard amount of exercise is an important fitness variable and the foundation for many CV endur-ance tests. There are many ways to assess HR both at rest and during exercise, including manually by palpation at various anatomic sites, use of an HR monitor, or with the electrocardiogram.

Measurement

HR can be measured by several techniques, during resting or exercise, including:

- Palpation of pulse at an anatomic site, such as the radial artery or carotid artery (the frequency of pulse waves per minute propagated along the peripheral arteries is usually identical to HR)
- Auscultation using a stethoscope to hear heart beat on chest (the lub-dub sound is equal to one contraction)
- HR monitor/watches
- Electrocardiography (the electrical waves of depolarization and repolarization of heart cells). Electro-cardiography is typically not used in health and fitness testing.

Palpation of Pulse There are two common anatomic sites for the measurement of HR:

- Radial: lightly press the index and middle fingers against the radial artery in the groove on the lateral wrist (bordered by the abductor pollicis longus and the extensor pollicis longus muscles). The radial palpation site is shown in Figure 2.8.
- Carotid: may be more visible or easily found than the radial pulse; press fingers lightly along the me-dial border of the sternocleidomastoid muscle in the lower neck (on either side). Avoid the carotid sinus area (stay well below their thyroid cartilage) to avoid the reflexive slowing of HR or drop in BP by the baroreceptor reflex. The carotid palpation site is shown in Figure 2.9.

If you experience difficulty in palpating the pulse, then use an HR monitor as a learning tool to check the palpated HR with the monitor's HR. All these methods, when applied correctly, will yield similar results. The palpation of the pulse method for HR measurement should be and can be mastered through practice. However, some clients, through anatomic differences, are more difficult to palpate.

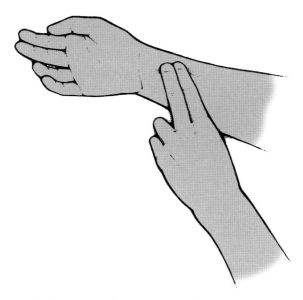

Figure 2.8 Radial artery site for heart rate measurement.

Norms for Resting Heart Rate Of note, measuring HR by palpation of the carotid artery may lead to an underestimation of the true HR. This is because the baroreceptors in the carotid sinus region become stimulated when touched. This may reflexively reduce the client's HR as the baroreceptors sense a false increase in BP. Therefore, the radial artery is the artery of choice for palpation. Perhaps the baroreceptor reflex becomes a more important issue with HR counts longer than 15 seconds. It is recommended that a full 60-second count be performed for accuracy in resting HR. However, a 30-second time period may be sufficient for the count. "Resting" conditions must be present (similar to resting BP). There are no known standards for resting HR classification.

Measurement of Exercise Heart Rate

By either palpation or auscultation, measure the number of beats felt or heard in a 10-, 15-, or 30-second period and multiply by 6 (10 seconds), 4 (15 seconds), or 2 (30 seconds) to convert to a 1-minute value (bpm). The 30-second count is more accurate and less prone to error than

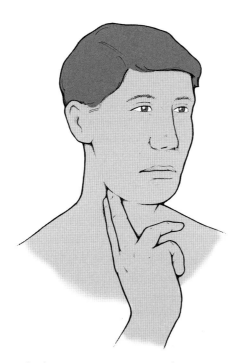

Figure 2.9 Carotid artery site for heart rate measurement.

a 15-second count. When counting the exercise HR for a time count period less than 1 minute, one should start the count at 0 (reference) at the first beat felt (or heard) and start the time period at that beat. Remember that the exercise HR is an extremely important variable for many CV endurance tests. The use of HR monitors has increased in popularity as these have become more available and affordable. Maximal exercise HR may be important for exercise prescription with the use of heart rate reserve (HRR) and $\dot{V}O_2$ reserve ($\dot{V}O_2R$) methods (see chapter 6) and for determining whether the exercise test is truly maximal and also a potential termination point for some submaximal cardiorespiratory exercise tests.

Rate Pressure Product

RPP, or DP, reflects myocardial (heart) oxygen demand or consumption (m$\dot{V}O_2$). RPP can be thought of as the heart's power output. The oxygen demand of the heart is related to the work of the heart. RPP is the product of HR and SBP.

$$RPP = (HR \times SBP) \times 10^{-2}$$

RPP is expressed in units where the resultant product is divided by 100 (10^{-2}) to better manage the integers.

For example:

If one's HR is 120 bpm with a BP of 150/90 mm Hg during submaximal exercise, then

$$RPP\ (m\dot{V}O_2) = (120 \times 150) \times 10^{-2} = 180$$

The RPP or m$\dot{V}O_2$ is useful in exercise testing and training of individuals with CVD. Often, a cardiac patient will experience angina, or chest pain, at a specific, replicable RPP or m$\dot{V}O_2$. Therefore, during exercise, if the cardiac patient exceeds a certain RPP (HR and SBP combination), he or she may experience angina. Thus, when prescribing exercise for these cardiac patients, one must consider their RPP to avoid the patients experiencing angina during their exercise.

BLOOD TESTS

To determine the presence of two of the coronary disease risk factors, lipids and blood glucose, a recent fasted blood test is required. Some clients who obtain regular physical examinations from their physician may have had a recent test. If so, this value can be used to determine the presence of risk factor. If the client does not recall the exact test values, a copy of the blood test report may need to be acquired from the health care provider.

Unfortunately, many American adults do not know their blood glucose and cholesterol values. Indeed, awareness in America regarding indicators and facts about diabetes and heart disease remains low. In 2009, the American Diabetes Association conducted a survey to test diabetes knowledge and concluded that "many Americans have very limited understanding of the basic facts about diabetes, as well as the serious consequences for health that accompany the disease" (15). Although one-third of the U.S. population has high cholesterol (16), awareness of cholesterol levels is lacking, and this is particularly true among specific subpopulations. For example, about one in five Latinos have high blood cholesterol, yet only half of those with this condition know it (17). Among women, a survey conducted by the Society for Women's Health Research reported that although 79% knew how much they weighed in high school, only 32% knew their cholesterol level (21% for 18- to 44-year-olds and 43% for 55 years and older) (18). The health risk assessment thus presents an opportunity to raise awareness of these risk factors and their implications on health.

The exercise professional has a few simple solutions if lipids and glucose values are unknown. First, a contract with a local laboratory that provides these blood testing services can be obtained and then clients can be referred to this facility for testing. Another option is to actually collect the blood sample from the client and then send the sample to the laboratory for analysis. A third option is to actually purchase the instrumentation for performing these tests. Many small, relatively economical systems are available commercially and offer the ability to perform lipids and glucose testing (and possibly other useful tests). Then, both collection and testing of the sample can be performed on-site. Generally, such results are available for interpretation within minutes.

Blood Sampling Methods

Phlebotomy is the practice of withdrawing blood from a blood vessel into a blood collection tube. Typically, this is done by either inserting a needle into a vein (larger volume sample) or puncturing a finger (smaller volume sample). The venipuncture method is obviously more involved and thus requires a skilled phlebotomist to perform the task. There are professional phlebotomy training courses available because this skill is needed in all medical facilities and can involve advanced skills, such as starting intravenous access lines, obtaining samples from arteries, and drawing samples from infants, children, and adults with characteristics that make the blood draw challenging. Fortunately, the sample needed for the cholesterol and glucose measures can be acquired by drawing a sample from a vein in the upper extremities. There are modified courses that can provide training limited to this purpose. Some states have regulations that restrict the practice of phlebotomy to those with a defined level of training; thus, the state department of health should be contacted to determine whether training and licensing regulations exist.

For facilities that purchase their own mini-sample systems, the blood sample can be obtained by a finger puncture, as shown in Figure 2.10. This skill is much simpler and requires less training. In most cases, an automated device is placed on the finger and then triggered to puncture the skin. Indeed, all individuals with diabetes are trained to perform this technique because they need to regularly self-monitor their blood glucose levels. The sample may be collected into a small capillary tube, or the drop of blood that forms on the finger may be applied directly to a reagent pad depending on the instrumentation used.

Standard Precautions

All health care and allied health care professionals should be trained to protect themselves against exposure to bloodborne pathogens. Indeed, the Occupational Safety and Health Administration of the Department of Labor has set national standards for these protections called *Standard Precautions*. A federal law (29 CFR 1910.1030) was first enacted in 1991 and provides the requirements for training and regular reviews of the procedures that should be followed to protect employees from the risks of exposure to bloodborne pathogens (19). Modifications to this law were further introduced in 2000 with The Needlestick Safety and Prevention Act (Pub L 106-430) (13). Certainly, all workers who will be involved in handling blood are required to have this training. However, it is reasonable for all exercise

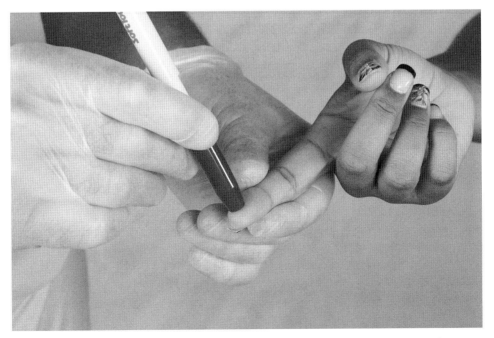

Figure 2.10 A device used to puncture the finger to obtain a blood sample. Note that protective gloves would be worn by the technician.

TABLE 2.4 • Classifications of Cholesterol and Triglyceride Levels (mg · dL⁻¹)

Non-HDL-C[a]	
<130	Desirable
130–159	Above desirable
160–189	Borderline high
190–219	High
≥220	Very high
LDL-C	
<100	Desirable
100–129	Above desirable
130–159	Borderline high
160–189	High
≥190	Very high
HDL-C	
<40 (men)	Low
<50 (women)	Low
Triglycerides	
<150	Normal
150–199	Borderline high
200–499	High
≥500	Very high[b]

[a]Non-HDL-C = Total cholesterol − HDL-C

[b]Severe hypertriglyceridemia is another term used for very high triglycerides in pharmaceutical product labeling.

HDL-C, high-density lipoprotein cholesterol; LDL-C, low-density lipoprotein cholesterol.

From Jellinger PS, Handelsman Y, Rosenblit PD, et al. American Association of Clinical Endocrinologists and American College of Endocrinology guidelines for management of dyslipidemia and prevention of cardiovascular disease. *Endocr Pract.* 2017;23(s2):1–87.

professionals who work with clients to assume that they may be at risk of exposure to blood (*e.g.*, an accident that results in a cut of the skin) or, possibly, other bodily fluids (with the exception of sweat). Thus, it is prudent for all exercise professionals to obtain training in standard precautions and be familiar with the laws regarding bloodborne pathogens.

Interpretation

Regardless of how the exercise professional obtains the blood test information, it is important to know how to interpret the results. The American Association of Clinical Endocrinologists and the American College of Endocrinology have standardized the interpretation of results of cholesterol, including HDL-C, low-density lipoprotein cholesterol (LDL-C), total cholesterol minus HDL-C (non-HDL-C), and triglycerides (Table 2.4) (8). Refer back to earlier in the chapter for the criteria for the positive risk factor of hypercholesterolemia and the negative risk factor of high HDL-C. Likewise, the American Diabetes Association has set the standards that have become uniformly accepted in health care for interpretation of fasting blood glucose (20). Prediabetes values are from 100 to 125 mg · dL⁻¹, values below 100 mg · dL⁻¹ are considered normal and values above 125 mg · dL⁻¹ are considered diagnostic for diabetes. Remember that as with resting BP, elevated values should be confirmed by at least one other test.

OBESITY

Obesity has been linked to an increased risk of various chronic conditions, including CVD, diabetes, several types of cancer, and musculoskeletal conditions (21). In fact, obesity is considered a major independent risk factor for the development of coronary artery disease (22,23).

Obesity is defined as an excessive amount of body fat. The assessment of body composition, which involves estimating body fat percentage, is the focus of Chapter 3 of this manual. From a risk factor assessment perspective, obesity is determined from evaluating an individual's body weight compared to his or her height and also considering the girth of the abdominal region of the body. The term *overweight* is used as classification for body weights that are above what is considered the normal range for one's height yet below the criteria for obesity.

Measurement of Height and Weight

Height is measured with an instrument called a *stadiometer*, which consists of a vertical ruler, is typically mounted to a wall, and has a sliding horizontal platform. When mounted to a wall, calibration becomes unnecessary because the measurement scale is fixed in place. Portable units and vertical rods attached to weight scales are also available; however, if these are used, then the stadiometer scale readings should be checked with a vertical ruler placed on the platform prior to each measurement session. Although height is a simple and relatively routine measurement to perform, the following important standardization steps as highlighted in Figure 2.11A and B should be used:

- The client must remove shoes and hat (if worn).
- The client should stand erect with feet flat on the floor with heels touching each other.
- If using a wall-mounted stadiometer, the heels, midbody, and upper body parts should be touching the wall.
- The client should inhale normally and hold it while looking straight ahead (head in a neutral position relative to the chin).
- The horizontal headboard should be lowered to touch the top of the head (skull).

Weight can be measured with various types of scales with different mechanisms. One of the most popular types is the balance beam scale. Regardless of the type of scale used, the accuracy of the mechanism should be checked regularly. Most scales provide a method to calibrate the zero point. Checking the scale with no weight on it is an essential step prior to each measurement. If the scale is not reading 0 as shown in Figure 2.12A, it should be adjusted to set the reading to 0 (Figure 2.12B). Some electronic scales also allow for a measurement of a standard amount of weight as a secondary check for accuracy. Ideally, this standard weight should be in the range of weights you expect for your clients; however, a

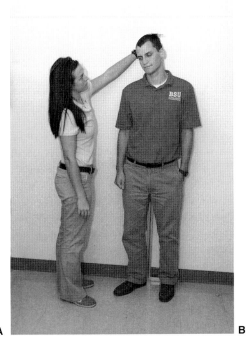
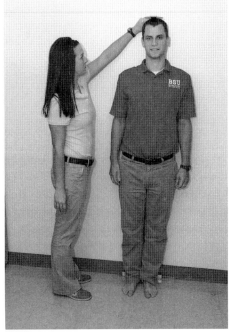

A   **B**

Figure 2.11 A: Incorrect technique used to measure height with a stadiometer; note that shoes are on, feet are not together, head is turned to the side, and the chin is tilted down. **B:** Correct standardized technique used to measure height with a stadiometer. Source: Photograph by Ball State University.

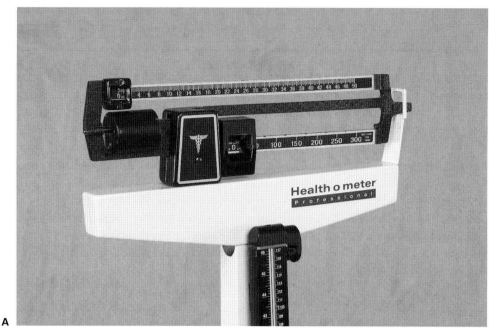

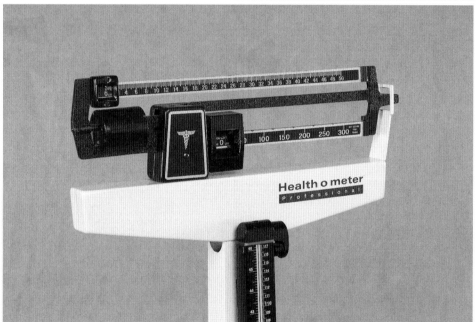

Figure 2.12 A: A scale needing calibration of the zero point. **B:** A correctly calibrated balance beam scale.

smaller amount of weight is commonly used because it is more practical. Some electronic scales may have the ability to adjust the scale if the standardized weight reading is deviant from the scale reading, thereby calibrating the scale at this weight. However, most scales do not have this second adjustment setting and will require professional service to restore accuracy. A calibration check log sheet, recording the date and zero and standard weight readings, should be kept by the exercise professional. Fortunately, most high-quality weight scales maintain their calibration quite well. The exercise professional still needs to regularly perform calibration checks to confirm the accuracy of clients' body weight readings. Like height, measuring weight is simple and relatively routine. To obtain accurate measurements, the following important standardization steps, as highlighted in Figure 2.13A and B, should be used:

- Clients should wear minimal clothing. In fitness assessment programs, this is generally considered shorts and a T-shirt (no shoes). However, in other settings with "street clothes," the client should be instructed to remove any outer layers and shoes, and also empty all pockets.
- The client should void the bladder prior (within 1 hour) to the measurement.

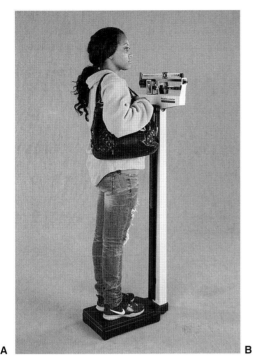 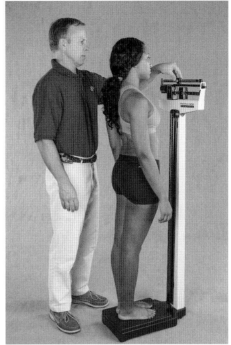

A   **B**

Figure 2.13 A: Incorrect technique used to measure weight; note that the shoes are on, and the patient is fully clothed and wearing a coat. **B:** Correct standardized technique used to measure weight.

- Ideally, weight should be measured in the morning prior to any meal or beverage consumption. However, because this is not always practical, the time of day should be similar for sequential measurement comparisons with no excess meal and beverage consumption prior to the measurement.

To track body weight over time, it is essential to follow the discussed standardizations. However, for screening programs, variations in the mentioned standards are acceptable with the understanding that the measured weight will be different from the standardized body weight.

Calculation of Body Mass Index

Body mass index (BMI), also called the Quetelet Index, is the weight-to-height ratio used to assess the obesity risk factor. This index compares an individual's weight (in kilograms) to his or her height (in meters squared). For example, an individual who weighs 165 lb and is 68 in tall would have a BMI calculated as follows:

Convert pounds to kilograms:	$165 \text{ lb}/2.2 \text{ lb} \cdot \text{kg}^{-1} = 74.8 \text{ kg}$
Convert inches to centimeters:	$68 \text{ in} \times 2.54 \text{ cm} \cdot \text{in}^{-1} = 172.7 \text{ cm}$
Convert centimeters to meters:	$172.7 \text{ cm}/100 \text{ cm} \cdot \text{m}^{-1} = 1.727 \text{ m}$
Square the meter measure:	$1.727 \text{ m} \times 1.727 \text{ m} = 2.98 \text{ m}^2$
Calculate BMI:	$74.8 \text{ kg}/2.98 \text{ m}^2 = 25.1 \text{ kg} \cdot \text{m}^{-2}$

Setting this formula up in a spreadsheet is a simple task and allows exercise professionals the ability to rapidly calculate BMI from height and weight measurements. In addition, there are many Web sites such as the one hosted by the Obesity Education Initiative of the National Heart, Lung, and Blood Institute that provide online calculators of BMI (24).

Measurement of Waist Circumference

The pattern of body weight distribution is recognized as an important predictor of health risks of obesity. Thus, the measurement of waist circumference is used as another indicator of obesity. This measurement identifies those with the abdominal type of obesity associated with greater health risk.

The waist circumference is typically measured at the smallest circumference above the umbilicus and below the xiphoid process. This measurement should be performed using the following important standardization steps as highlighted in Figure 2.14A and B:

- The technician should stand on the right side of the client.
- The measurement should be made on bare skin.

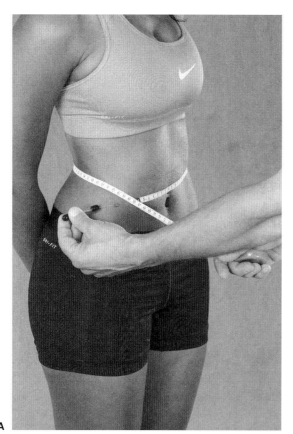

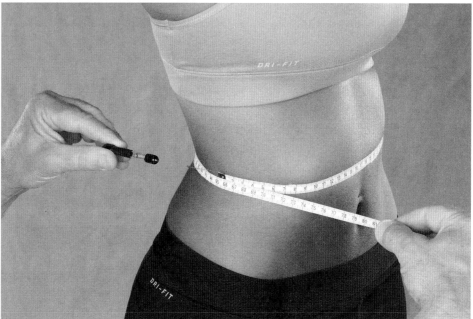

Figure 2.14 A: Incorrect technique used to measure waist circumference; note that the professional is standing in front of the client and the tape is not parallel to the floor. **B:** Correct standardized technique used to measure waist circumference.

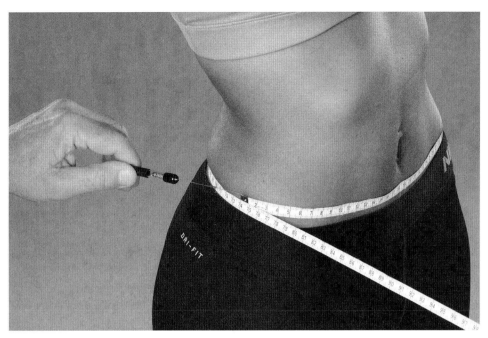

Figure 2.15 Measuring tape position for waist (abdominal) circumference using the alternative measurement site.

- The measurement should be taken at the end of a normal exhalation by the client.
- The measuring tape should be parallel to the floor and should be pulled to lay flat on the skin without compressing the skin (some measurement tapes have a gauge to standardize the tension).
- Multiple measurements should be taken to determine the smallest circumference site. The mean of two measurements at this location (that do not differ by more than 1 cm) is used.

An alternative measurement site was proposed by the National Obesity Task Force (NOTF). This site standardizes the location at horizontal measure directly above the iliac crest (Figure 2.15). Unfortunately, the NOTF does not provide any standardized formulas to be used (21).

Some have advocated the additional measurement of the hip circumference to assess body fat distribution. The two circumference values are used to determine the waist-to-hip ratio (WHR). The hip circumference is measured as the largest circumference around the buttocks, above the gluteal fold (posterior extension), following the same standardization procedures used for waist measurement.

Interpretation

The classifications for the obesity risk factor are provided earlier in the chapter. Note that either (not necessarily both) an elevated BMI ($\geq 30 \, \text{kg} \cdot \text{m}^{-2}$) or increased waist circumference (>88 cm for women or >102 cm for men) is used as the criterion for the obesity risk factor. Interestingly, one should be aware of two exceptions:

- There now appears to be some conflicting research regarding BMI risk classification within subpopulations of heart failure and AMI survivors. This phenomenon, known as the "obesity paradox," seems to show improved survival rates when BMI is $\geq 30 \, \text{kg} \cdot \text{m}^{-2}$, although the exact mechanism remains unclear (25,26).
- Asian populations develop health problems at lower BMI values in comparison to other population subgroups. Therefore, using lower cut points for defining overweight and obesity for Asian populations ($\geq 23.0 \, \text{kg} \cdot \text{m}^{-2}$ and $\geq 25.0 \, \text{kg} \cdot \text{m}^{-2}$, respectively) is recommended (27).

Additional classifications of BMI status and disease risk can be obtained using Table 2.5. In addition, further detail and information on other classifications for the waist circumference and the WHR are provided within *Chapter 3* of *ACSM's GETP11*.

TABLE 2.5 • Classification of Disease Risk Based on Body Mass Index (BMI) and Waist Circumference

| | | Disease Risk[a] Relative to Normal Weight and Waist Circumference | |
	BMI (kg · m^{-2})	Men ≤102 cm Women ≤88 cm	Men >102 cm Women >88 cm
Underweight	<18.5	—	—
Normal	18.5–24.9	—	—
Overweight	25.0–29.9	Increased	High
Obesity, class			
I	30.0–34.9	High	Very high
II	35.0–39.9	Very high	Very high
III	≥40.0	Extremely high	Extremely high

Dashes (—) indicate that no additional risk at these levels of BMI was assigned. Increased waist circumference can also be a marker for increased risk even in individuals of normal weight.

[a]Disease risk for type 2 diabetes, hypertension, and cardiovascular disease.

Modified from Executive summary of the clinical guidelines on the identification, evaluation, and treatment of overweight and obesity in adults. *Arch Intern Med.* 1998;158:1855–1867.

PHYSICAL ACTIVITY

PA represents one of the components of total daily energy expenditure, the other components being resting metabolic rate and the thermic effect of food. However, the voluntary nature of PA makes it the most variable component of total daily energy expenditure. Given the numerous health benefits of regular PA (28), public health guidelines have emerged regarding the recommended intensity and volume of PA necessary to promote health. Specifically, these guidelines advocate that long periods of inactivity should be avoided and that adults should obtain at least 150 minutes (2 hours and 30 minutes) a week of moderate-intensity or 75 minutes (1 hour and 15 minutes) a week of vigorous-intensity aerobic PA or an equivalent combination of moderate- and vigorous-intensity aerobic activities (28). The guidelines further state that these PA targets can be obtained by accumulating bouts of activity throughout the day in smaller increments, less than 10-minute durations. Given these recommendations, it is important to accurately assess the intensity, frequency, duration, and type of PA of an individual along with inactivity or sedentary time. This assessment becomes particularly critical when objectives involve refining the PA dose and health response relationship, investigating determinants to PA behavior, or evaluating intervention efforts to increase individual and population levels of PA. It is important to mention that regardless of the well-known health benefits of regular PA as described earlier, physical inactivity remains a global pandemic that has been identified as one of the four leading contributors to premature mortality (29,30).

From a risk assessment perspective, the highest interest lies in identifying those who are not meeting recommended amounts of PA (*i.e.*, inactive or irregularly active). Generally, the assessment of PA can be completed either through subjective assessment methods or via objective assessment methods.

Subjective Assessment

Subjective assessment methods include PA questionnaires, diaries, or logs. The level of detail can range from a four-item questionnaire attempting to distinguish overall global levels of activity (low vs. high levels) to a more detailed approach inquiring about different domains of activity (occupational, household, etc.) and the intensity, duration, frequency, and type of activity. There are many questionnaires that have been developed to assess PA.

The short version of the International Physical Activity Questionnaire (IPAQ), found in Box 2.5, is one that is relatively simple to use and can be completed by a client in about a minute (31). The instructions are straightforward, and the list of examples of PAs can be modified to fit the background of the client completing the questionnaire. The IPAQ uses a variable called metabolic equivalent

---

Box 2.5 International Physical Activity Questionnaire

We are interested in finding out about the kinds of physical activities that people do as part of their everyday lives. The questions will ask you about the time you spent being physically active in the **last 7 days**. Please answer each question even if you do not consider yourself to be an active person. Please think about the activities you do at work, as part of your house and yard work, to get from place to place, and in your spare time for recreation, exercise, or sport.

Think about all the **vigorous** activities that you did in the **last 7 days**.

Vigorous physical activities refer to activities that take hard physical effort and make you breathe much harder than normal.

Think *only* about those physical activities that you did for at least 10 minutes at a time.

1. During the **last 7 days**, on how many days did you do **vigorous** physical activities like heavy lifting, digging, aerobics, or fast bicycling?
   _____ **days per week** → How much time in total did you usually spend on one of these days doing vigorous physical activities?
   _____ **hours** _____ **minutes**
   or
   none
   Think about all the **moderate** activities that you did in the **last 7 days**. **Moderate** activities refer to activities that take moderate physical effort and make you breathe somewhat harder than normal. Think only about those physical activities that you did for at least 10 minutes at a time.
2. During the **last 7 days**, on how many days did you do **moderate** physical activities like carrying light loads, bicycling at a regular pace, or doubles tennis? Do not include walking.
   _____ **days per week** → How much time in total did you usually spend on one of these days doing moderate physical activities?
   _____ **hours** _____ **minutes**
   or
   none
   Think about the time you spent **walking** in the **last 7 days**.
   This includes walking at work and at home, walking to travel from place to place, and any other walking that you might do solely for recreation, sport, exercise, or leisure.
3. During the **last 7 days**, on how many days did you **walk** for at least 10 minutes at a time?
   _____ **days per week** → How much time in total did you usually spend on one of these days doing walking on one of those days?
   _____ **hours** _____ **minutes**
   or
   none
   The last question is about the time you spent **sitting** on weekdays during the **last 7 days**. Include time spent at work, at home, while doing course work and during leisure time. This may include time spent sitting at a desk, visiting friends, reading, or sitting or lying down to watch television.
4. During the **last 7 days**, how much time did you spend **sitting** on a **weekday**?
   _____ **hours** _____ **minutes**
   This is the end of the questionnaire, thank you.

From IPAQ. *International Physical Activity Questionnaire* [cited 2020 Jan 23]. Available from: https://docs.google.com/viewer?a=v&pid=sites&srcid=ZGVmYXVsdGRvbWFpbnx0aGVpcGFxfG-d4OjhlMTcxZGJkZmMxYTg1NQ (42).

(MET) · min · wk^{-1} for determining classifications. MET · min · wk^{-1} is calculated by multiplying the MET level for the type of activity by the number of minutes that activity was performed per day by the number of days per week the activity was performed. Walking is scored as 3.3 METs, moderate-intensity activities are scored as 4 METs, and vigorous-intensity activities are scored as 8 METs. For example, a person who reported performing moderate-intensity activity for 30 min · d^{-1} for 5 days of the week would have obtained 600 MET · min · wk^{-1} (4 METs $\times$ 30 min · d^{-1} $\times$ 5 d · wk^{-1}). PA-level classifications from the IPAQ assessment are presented in Table 2.6. It is important to recall that per Table 2.2, the criterion for defining the risk factor of physical inactivity *was not meeting the minimum threshold of 500 to 1,000 MET-minutes of moderate-to-vigorous PA, or 75 to 150 min · wk–^{1} of moderate- to vigorous-intensity PA.*

Objective Assessment

Objective assessment methods include assessment tools that are broadly defined as wearable devices (commercial wearable technology) and include motion sensors, HR monitoring, combination-type approaches (*i.e.*, accelerometer plus HR monitoring plus temperature), and global positioning system (GPS) tracking

TABLE 2.6 • Physical Activity Level Classifications from an International Physical Activity Questionnaire (IPAQ) Assessment	
Category 1 (low)	Not active enough to meet criteria for categories 2 or 3
Category 2 (moderate)	$\geq$3 d of vigorous activity of $\geq$20 min $\cdot$ d^{-1} OR $\geq$5 d of moderate-intensity activity or walking of $\geq$30 min $\cdot$ d^{-1} OR $\geq$5 d of any combination of walking or moderate- or vigorous-intensity activities achieving a minimum of 600 MET $\cdot$ min $\cdot$ wk^{-1}
Category 3 (high)	Vigorous-intensity activity $\geq$3 d $\cdot$ wk^{-1}, achieving at least 1500 MET $\cdot$ min $\cdot$ wk^{-1} OR 7 d of any combination of walking or moderate- or vigorous-intensity activities achieving a minimum of 3000 MET $\cdot$ min $\cdot$ wk^{-1}

From IPAQ. *International Physical Activity Scoring Protocol* [cited 2020 Jan 23]. Available from: https://sites. google.com/site/theipaq/scoring-protocol.

devices. Some types of monitors are typically worn on the body. For instance, pedometers/step counters and accelerometers can be worn at the level of the hip or ankle, HR monitors typically involve wearing an HR chest band and a watch-type receiver, and some combination monitors can be worn on the arm or at the hip. Manufacturers of these devices typically specify the chosen location to wear such devices. Objective monitors are usually small, lightweight, and unobtrusive. Alternatively, phone application may also be used to assess PA. Health and fitness phone applications have grown by about 330% between 2014 and 2017. Further, in 2016, 2017, and 2019, wearable devices were ranked as the top worldwide fitness trend (32,33).

The advantages and disadvantages of subjective and objective methods of assessing PA are outlined in Table 2.7. In choosing a PA assessment tool, be aware of the individual advantages and disadvantages of the method and match the tool chosen to the needs of the assessment. In most risk classification situations, it is advantageous to acquire immediate assessment of the client's PA behavior. In this instance, a paper questionnaire may be the tool of choice. However, with some advanced planning, objective monitors can be employed. Some facilities now offer assessments with accelerometers to obtain data on total inactivity time and time spent in light, moderate, and vigorous activities. Accelerometer reports can also provide information on bouts of moderate-to-vigorous intensity that last at least 10 minutes in duration. To capture the volatile nature of a person's PA with an objective assessment tool, a minimum period of observation is needed. It is recommended that these monitors be worn from the time the person wakes up in the morning until they go to bed at night. Assessing PA on both weekdays and weekends is recommended. More detailed information about several commercially available devices and accuracy has been reported elsewhere (34).

Interpretation

There can be numerous outcomes after assessing an individual's PA level, often dependent on the assessment method chosen. For instance, some activity questionnaires may display calories expended; others will output an index range of 1 to 4, with 1 being low active and 4 being the most active. Accelerometers may output the number of minutes a person spends being inactive and in light-, moderate-,

TABLE 2.7 • Comparison of Objective and Subjective Physical Activity Assessment Tools	Objective Assessment	Subjective Assessment
Advantages	Concurrent measure of activity — as one moves, it measures and records it Able to continuously record data for multiple days and weeks at a time Has an internal time clock, so activity can be time stamped to a specific time of day	Inexpensive Can be tailored to specific populations Can be administered to a large population
Disadvantages	Expensive Unable to determine type of activity May not capture nonambulatory activity (cycling, weightlifting)	Error from self-report (memory) and self-perception (intensity) Poor in assessing typical activities of daily living (*i.e.*, lifestyle activities)

TABLE 2.8 • Classification of Physical Activity Behavior	
Inactive	No activity beyond baseline activities of daily living.
Low activity	Activity beyond baseline but fewer than 150 min (2 h and 30 min) of moderate-intensity physical activity a week or the equivalent amount (75 min or 1 h and 15 min) of vigorous-intensity physical activity
Medium activity	150–300 (5 h) min of moderate-intensity physical activity a week (or 75–150 min of vigorous-intensity physical activity a week). In scientific terms, this range is approximately equivalent to 500–1000 metabolic equivalent (MET) minutes a week.
High activity	More than the equivalent of 300 min of moderate-intensity physical activity a week

or vigorous-intensity activity on a daily basis, whereas a pedometer/step counter will yield the total number of steps taken on a particular day. GPS tracking devices can track the number of variables per individual workout, such as HR, caloric expenditure, and the number of steps. Many of these output units are not interchangeable, or they become less valid in conversion. For instance, an attempt to convert steps accumulated per day into calories expended per day will result in the loss of some measurement accuracy. The validity of the method chosen and the selected output variable should always be considered when measuring PA levels.

Interpreting an individual's PA level can establish a profile of behavior and classify the person as either engaging in enough activity to be health enhancing or engaging in too little activity and being classified as sedentary or inactive. Seasonal variation is also evident in PA behavior and needs to be considered when assessing and comparing PA patterns. Table 2.8 presents a classification system of PA behavior.

SUMMARY

Preassessment screening includes informed consent and determination of the recommendations for medical clearance before performing the fitness assessment. The informed consent is a process that involves several key elements, allowing the client to completely understand the essential factors related to performing the fitness assessment. The determination of the need for medical clearance helps the exercise professional guide the client in making decisions about health readiness to proceed with the fitness assessment. Many exercise professionals can provide a valuable service by offering measurements of several different factors related to risk classification assessment. These additional measurements do require specialized training and some instrumentation. Minimally, the exercise professional should know resources in the community where these services can be obtained and needs to be knowledgeable about the interpretation of the results from these risk factor assessments.

LABORATORY ACTIVITIES

Readiness Assessment Using ACSM's Exercise Preparticipation Health Screening Questionnaire for Exercise Professionals (Figure 2.3)

Data Collection

With a relative older than 45 years of age, complete the questionnaire (be sure to omit a name or any identifying information with your assignment). Review the questionnaire with this individual.

Written Report

Determine whether this person is presented with any sign or symptoms suggestive of CV, metabolic, or renal diseases.

Evaluation of Medications Before Participation in a Physical Fitness Evaluation

Data Collection

Ask a friend or relative older than 55 years of age who is presently taking three or more medications to provide you with a complete list of the names of each medication along with the dosage and frequency of use (be sure to omit a name or any identifying information with your assignment).

Written Report

Provide a summary of the following for each medication:
- The reason the person is taking the medication (*i.e.*, the indication for use)
- The common side effects of the medication
- The potential for this medication effecting the person's response to exercise, especially note if the medication may change the person's HR

Administering an Informed Consent

In-Class Project

With a laboratory partner, practice verbally reviewing the key elements of an informed consent and providing an explanation of procedures for a body composition assessment.

Resting Blood Pressure and Heart Rate Assessments

Data Collection

- Perform a calibration check of the aneroid manometer you will use for the laboratory. Record the results of this calibration check and provide an interpretation.
- Measure eight students' resting BP and allow eight students to measure your resting BP following the procedures in Box 3.2. Record the values that were measured on you below (do not let the technician see the previous measurement values).

Technician	1	2	3	4	5	6	7	8
SBP								
DBP								
HR								

Written Report

1. Graph the data and comment on the variability in the measurements. Provide a critique of any deviations from recommended techniques you observed from watching the technicians. Using the mean values for SBP, DBP, and HR, provide an interpretation of your resting BP and HR.
2. Provide responses for the following:
   - Describe the white coat syndrome.
   - Explain how the principle of the auscultatory method is used for BP assessment.
   - Which of the Korotkoff sounds is used for SBP? What phase of the Korotkoff sounds is *true* DBP?

Body Mass Index Assessment

Data Collection

- Measure eight students' height, weight, and waist circumference and allow eight students to make these measures on you following the procedures in this manual. Record the values that were measured on you below (do not let the technician see the previous measurement values). Calculate the BMI (show your work on these calculations).

Technician	1	2	3	4	5	6	7	8
Height								
Weight								
BMI								
Waist								

Written Report

1. Graph the data and comment on the variability in the measurements. Provide a critique of any deviations from recommended techniques you observed from watching the technicians.
2. Using the mean values for height, weight, and waist circumference, provide an interpretation of your BMI and disease risk.

International Physical Activity Questionnaire Assessment

Data Collection

- Complete a short-form IPAQ (Box 2.5).
- Ask two friends or relatives (one of each gender) who work full time to complete a short-form IPAQ.

Written Report

1. Perform the calculations of $MET \cdot min \cdot wk^{-1}$ on each of these three PA assessments.
2. Provide interpretations of each of the three subjects' IPAQ PA classifications and explain the criteria you used to choose the classification category.

REFERENCES

1. Department of Health and Human Services. Health Insurance Portability and Accountability (HIPPA) Act 1996; [cited 2020 Jan 23]. Available from: https://www.gpo.gov/fdsys/pkg/PLAW-104publ191/pdf/PLAW-104publ191.pdf.
2. HHS.gov Health Information Technology for Economic and Clinical Health Act of 2009; [cited 2018 Jan 10] Available online: https://www hhs gov/hipaa/for-professionals/special-topics/hitech-act-enforcement-interim-final-rule/index html.
3. American College of Sports Medicine. *ACSM's Guidelines for Exercise Testing and Prescription*. 11th ed. Philadelphia (PA): Wolters Kluwer; 2021.
4. Magal M, Riebe D. New preparticipation health screening recommendations: what exercise professionals need to know. *ACSM's Health Fitness J.* 2016;20(3):22–7.
5. Roger VL, Go AS, Lloyd-Jones DM, et al. Executive summary: heart disease and stroke statistics — 2012 update: a report from the American Heart Association. *Circulation.* 2012;125(1):188-97.
6. Thompson PD, Baggish AL, Franklin B, Jaworski C, Riebe D. American College of Sports Medicine Expert Consensus Statement to Update Recommendations for Screening, Staffing, and Emergency Policies to Prevent Cardiovascular Events at Health Fitness Facilities. *Curr Sports Med Rep.* 2020;19(6):223–31.
7. Myers J, Forman DE, Balady GJ, et al. Supervision of exercise testing by nonphysicians: a scientific statement from the American Heart Association. *Circulation.* 2014;130(12):1014-27.
8. Jellinger PS, Handelsman Y, Rosenblit PD, et al. American Association of Clinical Endocrinologists and American College of Endocrinology guidelines for management of dyslipidemia and prevention of cardiovascular disease. *Endocr Pract.* 2017;23(s2):1-87.
9. Arnett DK, Blumenthal RS, Albert MA, et al. 2019 ACC/AHA Guideline on the Primary Prevention of Cardiovascular Disease. *A Report of the American College of Cardiology/American Heart Association Task Force on Clinical Practice Guidelines. J Am Coll Cardiol.* 2019;74(10):e177-232. doi:10.1016/j.jacc.2019.03.010.
10. U.S. National Library of Medicine. Drug information Portal [Internet]. 2020 [cited 2020 Jan 31]. Available from: https://druginfo.nlm.nih.gov/drugportal/.
11. Pickering TG, Hall JE, Appel LJ, et al. Recommendations for blood pressure measurement in humans and experimental animals: part 1: blood pressure measurement in humans: a statement for professionals from the Subcommittee of Professional and Public Education of the American Heart Association Council on High Blood Pressure Research. *Hypertension.* 2005;45(1):142-61.

12. United States Environmental Protection Agency. Mercury. 2020 [cited 2020 Jan 31]. Available from: https://www.epa.gov/mercury#facilities.

13. Tatelbaum FM. Needlestick safety and prevention act. *Pain Physician*. 2001;4(2):193-5.

14. Whelton PK, Carey RM, Aronow WS, et al. 2017 ACC/AHA/AAPA/ABC/ACPM/AGS/APhA/ASH/ASPC/NMA/PCNA guideline for the prevention, detection, evaluation, and management of high blood pressure in adults: a report of the American College of Cardiology/American Heart Association Task Force on Clinical Practice Guidelines. *J Am Coll Cardiol*. 2018;71(19):e127-248.

15. American Diabetes Association. As America earns failing grade, American Diabetes Association launches movement to stop diabetes. *American Diabetes Association Survey Finds* [Internet]. 2009 [cited 2011 July 15]. Available from: http://www.diabetes.org/for-media/2009/america-earns-failing-adm-sd-2009.html.

16. Benjamin EJ, Blaha MJ, Chiuve SE, et al. Heart disease and stroke statistics-2017 update: a report from the American Heart Association. *Circulation*. 2017;135(10):e146-603.

17. U.S. Department of Health and Human Services. Do you know your cholesterol levels? Healthy hearts, healthy homes. 2008 [cited 2020 Jan 23]. Available from: https://www.nhlbi.nih.gov/files/docs/public/heart/cholesterol.pdf.

18. Smith SC, Allen J, Blair SN, et al. AHA/ACC guidelines for secondary prevention for patients with coronary and other atherosclerotic vascular disease: 2006 update: endorsed by the National Heart, Lung, and Blood Institute. *J Am Coll Cardiol*. 2006;47(10):2130-9.

19. United States Department of Labor. Bloodborne pathogens. 1992 [cited 2020 Jan 23]. Available from: https://www.osha.gov/pls/oshaweb/owadisp.show_document?p_id=10051&p_table=STANDARDS.

20. American Diabetes Association. Classification and diagnosis of diabetes: standards of medical care in diabetes — 2019. *Diabetes Care*. 2019;42(Supplement 1):S13-28.

21. National Heart, Lung, and Blood Institute. *Clinical Guidelines on the Identification, Evaluation, and Treatment of Overweight and Obesity in Adults: The Evidence Report*. Bethesda (MD): National Heart, Lung, and Blood Institute; 1998.

22. Eckel RH, Krauss RM. American Heart Association call to action: obesity as a major risk factor for coronary heart disease. *Circulation*. 1998;97(21):2099-100.

23. Expert Panel on the Identification, Evaluation, and Treatment of Overweight and Obesity in Adults. Executive summary of the clinical guidelines on the identification, evaluation, and treatment of overweight and obesity in adults. *Arch Intern Med*. 1998;158:1855-67.

24. National Heart, Lung, and Blood Institute. Calculate your body mass index; [cited 2020 Jan 23]. Available from: http://www.nhlbi.nih.gov/health/educational/lose_wt/BMI/bmicalc.htm.

25. Arena R, Lavie CJ. The obesity paradox and outcome in heart failure: is excess bodyweight truly protective? *Future Cardiol*. 2010;6(1):1-6.

26. Bucholz EM, Beckman AL, Krumholz HA, Krumholz HM, Dr. Bucholz was affiliated with the Yale School of Medicine and Yale School of Public Health during the time that the work was conducted. Excess weight and life expectancy after acute myocardial infarction: the obesity paradox reexamined. *Am Heart J*. 2016;172:173-81.

27. Hsu WC, Araneta MRG, Kanaya AM, Chiang JL, Fujimoto W. BMI cut points to identify at-risk Asian Americans for type 2 diabetes screening. *Diabetes Care*. 2015;38(1):150-8.

28. Physical Activity Guidelines for Americans. 2018 physical activity guidelines advisory committee scientific report. U.S. Department of Health and Human Services; 2018. Available from: https://health.gov/sites/default/files/2019-09/PAG_Advisory_Committee_Report.pdf

29. Hallal PC, Andersen LB, Bull FC, et al. Global physical activity levels: surveillance progress, pitfalls, and prospects. *Lancet*. 2012;380(9838):247-57.

30. Kohl 3rd HW, Craig CL, Lambert EV, et al. The pandemic of physical inactivity: global action for public health. *Lancet*. 2012;380(9838):294-305.

31. International Physical Activity Questionnaire. IPAQ Scoring Protocol. 2005 [cited 2020 Jan 23]. Available from: https://sites.google.com/site/theipaq/scoring-protocol.

32. Thompson WR. Worldwide survey of fitness trends for 2019. *ACSM's Health Fitness J*. 2018;22(6):10-7.

33. Netimperative. Health and fitness app usage "grew 330% in just 3 years." 2017 [cited 2020 April 27]. Available from: http://www.netimperative.com/2017/09/13/health-fitness-app-usage-grew-330-just-3-years/.

34. Bunn JA, Navalta JW, Fountaine CJ, Reece JD. Current state of commercial wearable technology in physical activity monitoring 2015–2017. *Int J Exerc Sci*. 2018;11(7):503.

35. Gibbons RJ, Balady GJ, Bricker JT, et al. ACC/AHA 2002 guideline update for exercise testing: summary article: a report of the American College of Cardiology/American Heart Association Task Force on Practice Guidelines (Committee to Update the 1997 Exercise Testing Guidelines). *J Am Coll Cardiol*. 2002;40(8):1531-40.

36. Mozaffarian D, Benjamin EJ, Go AS, et al. Executive summary: heart disease and stroke statistics — 2015 update: a report from the American Heart Association. *Circulation*. 2015;131(4):434-41.

37. Verrill D, Graham H, Vitcenda M, Peno-Green L, Kramer V, Corbisiero T. Measuring behavioral outcomes in cardiopulmonary rehabilitation: an AACVPR statement. *J Cardiopulm Rehabil Prev*. 2009;29(3):193-203.

38. Jensen MD, Ryan DH, Apovian CM, et al. 2013 AHA/ACC/TOS guideline for the management of overweight and obesity in adults: a report of the American College of Cardiology/American Heart Association Task Force on Practice Guidelines and The Obesity Society. *J Am Coll Cardiol*. 2014;63(25 Part B):2985-3023.

39. Arnett DK, Blumenthal RS, Albert MA, et al. 2019 ACC/AHA guideline on the primary prevention of cardiovascular disease: executive summary: a report of the American College of Cardiology/American Heart Association Task Force on Clinical Practice Guidelines. *J Am Coll Cardiol*. 2019;74(10):1376-414.

40. Fletcher GF, Ades PA, Kligfield P, et al. Exercise standards for testing and training: a scientific statement from the American Heart Association. *Circulation*. 2013;128(8):873-934.

41. Kantola I, Vesalainen R, Kangassalo K, Kariluoto A. Bell or diaphragm in the measurement of blood pressure? *J Hypertens*. 2005;23(3):499-503.

42. International Physical Activity Questionnaire. Self-administered, short-form. 2002 [cited 2020 Jan 23]. Available from: https://docs.google.com/viewer?a=v&pid=sites&srcid=ZGVmYXVsdGRvbWFpbnx0aGVpcGFxfGd4OjhlMTcxZGJkZm-MxYTg1NQ.

Body Composition

WHY MEASURE BODY COMPOSITION

In the most general sense, body composition is the study of the components of the body and their relative proportions, and there is clinical value to knowing the amount of these varied components. For example, the total amount (mass) and density of bone tissue is a critical measure to assess in the diagnosis and prognosis of osteoporosis. From a fitness assessment point of view, *body composition* is defined as the relative proportions of fat and fat-free tissue in the body, usually expressed as a total body fat percentage. Typically, the focus of a body composition assessment is to obtain an estimate of body fat percentage or to determine the amount, or percentage, of muscle mass. Some of the more common uses of body composition assessments include the following:

- Identifying health risks, or promoting understanding of health risks, associated with too little or too much body fat
- Assessing the effectiveness of exercise and/or nutrition interventions

- Estimating ideal body weight to formulate dietary recommendations and exercise prescriptions
- Monitoring growth, development, maturation, and age-related changes in body composition, especially in children
- Formulating interventions to prevent chronic diseases later in life

Health Implications

In Chapter 2, the risks of obesity, as measured by body mass index (BMI) and waist circumference, were discussed. As a result of the high prevalence of obesity, many fitness professionals emphasize body composition assessment to their clients. However, obesity is not the singular concern of health and fitness professionals because too low levels of body fat also merit recognition for its associated health risks. This is particularly relevant in certain populations where individuals are at greater risk for developing eating disorders and all athletes who are involved in sports where weight is thought to impact performance (1). Unless clinically indicated, the assessment of body composition is typically not recommended for those with or at risk for developing an eating disorder.

It is also important to recognize changes in body composition that accompany aging. *Sarcopenia* is defined as loss of muscle mass, with accompanying decreases in strength, which is due to the aging process and reduced physical activity (2). Although precise measurement of the total amount of muscle mass is not obtained in a body composition assessment, it is a major component of the fat-free tissue that is estimated and as such should be reported. Indeed, it is important to recognize that it is the muscle mass that is most directly related to both muscular and cardiorespiratory fitness.

Functional Implications

Both obesity and sarcopenia can result in some degree of functional impairment, which may include decreased walking speed, stability, postural control, and neurocognitive function and increases in musculoskeletal pain. Although younger individuals often do not recognize the association between excess body weight and these conditions, their risk is just as real. In fact, because the prevalence of obesity among children and youth increased substantially over the past few years in the United States (3), there is an increased likelihood that these impairments will be more common and begin to occur early in the life span. Explaining and discussing the functional limitations of obesity may be key in promoting an understanding of the negative effects of obesity. Such a discussion may subsequently encourage involvement in a fitness program.

Many adults rarely perform activities that require high levels of muscular power, and most have neglected any form of resistance exercise training, thereby making the onset of sarcopenia more likely and at an earlier age. Sarcopenia is also identified as a major predictor of disability, which then leads to nursing home institutionalization regardless of age (4). Thus, muscle mass estimates should be considered a key component of a fitness assessment in adults, particularly those with a sparse physical activity background, because the assessment may provide sufficient motivation to incorporate muscular fitness training into an individual's exercise programs.

WHAT IS THE GOLD STANDARD TEST?

There is no one method that exists to accurately quantify the total amount of body fat in a living individual. Some clinical measures, as discussed in the next section, can provide accurate determinations of the amount of body fat in particular segments of the body. However, more investigations are needed prior to applying these expensive technologies in the determination of total body fat percentage.

Historically, the method of underwater (hydrostatic) weighing has been considered a gold standard for body fat percentage assessments. This method, used to determine body density (Db), has typically been employed as the standard against which other methods are compared. An overview of underwater weighing is provided later in this chapter. It is important to keep in mind that prior to beginning any assessment, it is important that the participant has provided consent and, at a minimum, a Physical Activity Readiness Questionnaire for Everyone (PAR-Q+) has been provided as a screening tool.

CLINICAL MEASURES

Fitness professionals will have limited ability to obtain true clinical measures of body composition for their clients. However, some clients may obtain these measures as part of their medical care and may bring the results to the fitness professional for advice.

Magnetic Resonance Imaging and Computed Tomography

Magnetic resonance imaging (MRI) and computed tomography (CT) scans are typically used as diagnostic procedures for various diseases. These devices take a cross-sectional picture (think of this as one thin slice) of a particular body region and produce an image allowing for a precise look at the fat and fat-free mass. These technologies can assess the change in the amount of fat, bone, and muscle tissue related to different interventions, including exercise. Figure 3.1 shows an MRI scan of a segment of the thighs of a 30-year-old woman. Figure 3.2 shows a CT scan of a segment of the abdomen in an older man. Note the layer of subcutaneous fat on both of these scans. In an experimental research study, scans will be taken at the same location before and after an intervention, allowing for any changes to be accurately measured in each distinct segment of the body.

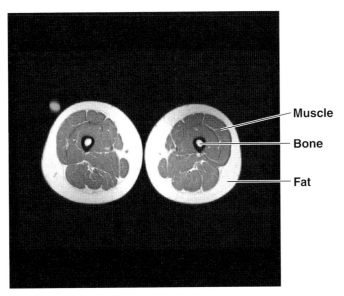

Figure 3.1 A magnetic resonance imaging scan of the thighs of a 30-year-old woman. Source: Ball State University — Dr. Todd Trappe.

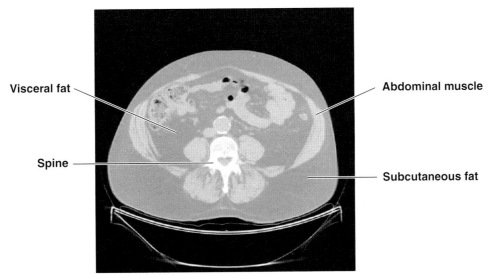

Figure 3.2 A computed tomography scan of the abdomen of an older man. Source: Ball State University — Dr. Todd Trappe.

Dual-Energy X-Ray Absorptiometry

Dual-energy X-ray absorptiometry (DXA) measurements are ordered for individuals as a diagnostic test for osteoporosis, with the main outcome measure being bone density. However, X-ray technology today allows for the assessment of the relative amounts of other body components such as fat and lean tissue. Therefore, another valuable feature of DXA is its ability to evaluate regional body fat proportions, which can be remeasured over time to identify changes. Figure 3.3 shows an example of one total body DXA scan and the body composition report.

TESTS OF BODY VOLUME

The measurement of volume is used to determine density using the following formula:

$$\text{Density} = \text{mass/volume}$$

Different types of body tissues have different density values. In body composition assessments, the known difference in the density of fat versus fat-free tissues is used to derive estimates of body

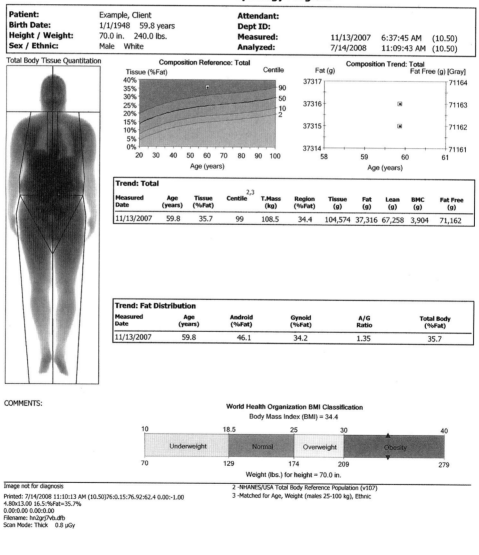

Figure 3.3 A body composition report from a total body dual-energy X-ray absorptiometry scan. Source: Ball State University—Clinical Exercise Physiology Program.

Ball State University
Human Performance Laboratory
Clinical Exercise Physiology Program

Patient:	Example, Client		Attendant:			
Birth Date:	1/1/1948 59.8 years		Dept ID:			
Height / Weight:	70.0 in. 240.0 lbs.		Measured:	11/13/2007 6:37:45 AM (10.50)		
Sex / Ethnic:	Male White		Analyzed:	7/14/2008 11:09:43 AM (10.50)		

BODY COMPOSITION

Region	Tissue (%Fat)	Region (%Fat)	Tissue (g)	Fat (g)	Lean (g)	BMC (g)	Total Mass (kg)
Left Arm	26.0	24.8	5,264	1,371	3,893	260	-
Left Leg	31.8	30.4	15,430	4,904	10,526	714	-
Left Trunk	41.4	40.4	28,830	11,923	16,908	684	-
Left Total	35.6	34.4	52,680	18,780	33,900	1,981	-
Right Arm	26.0	24.9	5,314	1,383	3,931	252	-
Right Leg	31.8	30.5	15,511	4,935	10,575	688	-
Right Trunk	41.4	40.4	28,294	11,706	16,588	708	-
Right Total	35.7	34.4	51,894	18,536	33,358	1,923	-
Arms	26.0	24.8	10,578	2,754	7,824	512	-
Legs	31.8	30.4	30,941	9,839	21,102	1,402	-
Trunk	41.4	40.4	57,125	23,628	33,496	1,393	-
Android	46.1	45.7	10,249	4,720	5,529	84	-
Gynoid	34.2	33.3	15,827	5,414	10,413	416	-
Total	35.7	34.4	104,574	37,316	67,258	3,904	108.5

FAT MASS RATIOS

Trunk/ Total	Legs/ Total	(Arms+Legs)/ Trunk
0.63	0.26	0.53

3 -Matched for Age, Weight (males 25-100 kg), Ethnic

B   GE Healthcare

Lunar Prodigy
DF+10199

Figure 3.3 (*Continued*)

fat percentage. Mass, or body weight, can be accurately determined following the procedures outlined in Chapter 3. Two widely used body volume assessment methods—underwater weighing and plethysmography — allow for the determination of body volume. Each of these methods is discussed in detail in the next section. Once volume has been derived, Db is then used to estimate body fat percentage.

Individuals with different characteristics typically have different Db; therefore, population-specific equations have been developed to determine body fat (see Table 3.1). These equations were developed around the knowledge that body mass can be differentiated based on two components: fat mass and fat-free mass, and it is not without its limitations (2).

Hydrostatic (Underwater) Weighing

The hydrostatic weighing method for determining body volume is based on Archimedes principle, which states that a body immersed in a fluid is buoyed up by a force equal to the weight of the fluid displaced. Therefore, hydrostatic weighing measures body volume via water displacement. To determine body volume via hydrostatic weighing requires measurements of body weight before entering the water

TABLE 3.1 • Population-Specific Formulas for Conversion of Body Density to Percent Body Fat

	Population	Age (Years)	Sex	%BF[a]	FFBd[b] (g · cm⁻³)
Ethnicity	African American	9–17	Women	$(5.24/Db) - 4.82$	1.088
		19–45	Men	$(4.85/Db) - 4.39$	1.106
		24–79	Women	$(4.86/Db) - 4.39$	1.106
	American Indian	18–62	Men	$(4.97/Db) - 4.52$	1.099
		18–60	Women	$(4.81/Db) - 4.34$	1.108
	Asian Japanese Native	18–48	Men	$(4.97/Db) - 4.52$	1.099
			Women	$(4.76/Db) - 4.28$	1.111
		61–78	Men	$(4.87/Db) - 4.41$	1.105
			Women	$(4.95/Db) - 4.50$	1.1
	Singaporean (Chinese, Indian, Malay)		Men	$(4.94/Db) - 4.48$	1.102
			Women	$(4.84/Db) - 4.37$	1.107
	Caucasian	8–12	Men	$(5.27/Db) - 4.85$	1.086
			Women	$(5.27/Db) - 4.85$	1.086
		13–17	Men	$(5.12/Db) - 4.69$	1.092
			Women	$(5.19/Db) - 4.76$	1.09
		18–59	Men	$(4.95/Db) - 4.50$	1.1
			Women	$(4.96/Db) - 4.51$	1.101
		60–90	Men	$(4.97/Db) - 4.52$	1.099
			Women	$(5.02/Db) - 4.57$	1.098
	Hispanic		Men	NA	NA
		20–40	Women	$(4.87/Db) - 4.41$	1.105
Athletes	Resistance trained	24 ± 4	Men	$(5.21/Db) - 4.78$	1.089
		35 ± 6	Women	$(4.97/Db) - 4.52$	1.099
	Endurance trained	21 ± 2	Men	$(5.03/Db) - 4.59$	1.097
		21 ± 4	Women	$(4.95/Db) - 4.50$	1.1
	All sports	18–22	Men	$(5.12/Db) - 4.68$	1.093
		18–22	Women	$(4.97/Db) - 4.52$	1.099
Clinical populations[c]	Anorexia nervosa	15–44	Women	$(4.96/Db) - 4.51$	1.101
	Cirrhosis				
	Childs A			$(5.33/Db) - 4.91$	1.084
	Childs B			$(5.48/Db) - 5.08$	1.078
	Childs C			$(5.69/Db) - 5.32$	1.07
	Obesity	17–62	Women	$(4.95/Db) - 4.50$	1.1
	Spinal cord injury (paraplegic/quadriplegic)	18–73	Men	$(4.67/Db) - 4.18$	1.116
		18–73	Women	$(4.70/Db) - 4.22$	1.114

[a]Multiply by 100 for percentage of body fat.

[b]Fat-free body density (FFBd) based on average values reported in selected research articles.

[c]There are insufficient multicomponent model data to estimate the average FFBd of the following clinical populations: coronary artery disease, heart/lung transplants, chronic obstructive pulmonary disease, cystic fibrosis, diabetes mellitus, thyroid disease, human immunodeficiency virus (HIV)/acquired immunodeficiency syndrome (AIDS), cancer, kidney failure (dialysis), multiple sclerosis, and muscular dystrophy.

%BF, percentage of body fat; Db, body density; NA, no data available for this population subgroup.

Adapted with permission from Heyward VH, Wagner DR. *Applied Body Composition Assessment*. 2nd ed. Champaign (IL): Human Kinetics; 2004. p. 9.

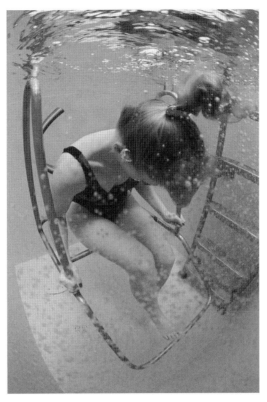

Figure 3.4 The underwater weighing procedure.

and then measuring the loss of body weight when submerged underwater, hence the term "underwater weighing" (Figure 3.4). The underwater weight is influenced by two separate amounts of air trapped in the body: residual lung volume and gas in the gastrointestinal (GI) system. These components of trapped air contribute to buoyancy and thus need to be factored into the calculation of underwater weight. Ideally, residual volume should be directly measured; however, it is often predicted. GI gas is calculated as a constant value of 100 mL. The following common formulas are used to estimate residual volume based on sex, height (cm), and age (years) (5,6):

Men:Residual volume $(L) = [0.019 \times \text{height (cm)}] + [0.0155 \times \text{age (years)}] - 2.24$ (1)

Women:Residual volume $(L) = [0.032 \times \text{height (cm)}] + [0.009 \times \text{age (years)}] - 3.90$ (7)

Plethysmography

As with hydrostatic weighing, plethysmography is also based on the concept of displacement, but in this procedure, the matter being displaced is air. A body plethysmograph can determine changes in volume (V) with measures of pressure (P) according to Boyle law ($P_1V_1 = P_2V_2$, if temperature is constant). One manufacturer, COSMED*, sells a whole-body plethysmograph (the BOD POD) to provide measures of body volume by assessing air displacement. The BOD POD plethysmograph contains two separate chambers used to measure air displacement. Measurements of pressure and volume are made through three consecutive measures: first with the front chamber empty, then with a standard cylinder of known volume to calibrate the system, and finally with a person in the front chamber. The second chamber, or back chamber, remains closed at all times and simply serves as a reference chamber. This procedure requires the client to follow similar pretest standardizations as for underwater weighing (see Box 3.1). In addition, the client must wear only tight-fitting clothing made of nylon (typically, a swimsuit or cycling shorts and a sports bra) and a swim cap to control for temperature variations caused by hair on the head, as shown in Figure 3.5. The client only needs to remain still while the instrument measures body volume, thus making this procedure less demanding and less time-consuming than underwater weighing. The outcome measure of body volume is then used to calculate Db.

Box 3.1	Procedures for Underwater Weighing

Pretest Standardizations

1. Clients should be in a normally hydrated state and should not have eaten for at least 3 hours.
2. Immediately prior to the assessment, clients should empty the bladder and attempt to empty the bowels.
3. Clients should remove any makeup, body oils, and jewelry prior to entering the water.
4. Clients should wear a tight-fitting swimsuit to eliminate air trapping.
5. Explain to clients that they should begin exhaling as they gently submerge themselves under the water and to continue exhaling as much as possible. At that point, they need to remain underwater as long as possible and remain as still as possible to obtain a stable underwater weight reading. This procedure will need to be repeated multiple times (typically, 5–10) because there is generally a learning effect for this procedure.

Assessment Procedures

1. Obtain a body weight measurement on clients before they enter the water.
2. Measure the temperature of the water.
3. Have clients enter the water and sit on the suspended chair.
4. Have clients submerge themselves underwater, following the instructions provided. Note that some clients may require that the chair be weighted if while performing the procedure, a part of their body breaks the surface of the water (because of buoyancy).
5. Repeat Step 4 until at least three consecutive underwater weight readings do not increase.

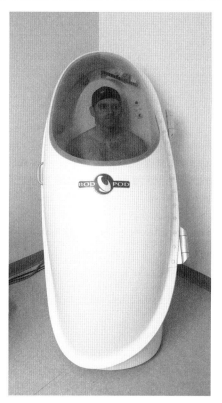

Figure 3.5 A client having his body fat percentage estimated using whole-body plethysmography.

ANTHROPOMETRY

Anthropometry is the measurement of the human body, which includes measures of height, weight, and BMI, as mentioned in Chapter 2, and skinfolds as well as circumferences or girths. Anthropometric measurements are made at various specific sites on the body.

Skinfold Measurements

Skinfold measurements can be used to estimate body fat percentage based on the assumption that the amount of subcutaneous fat is proportional to the total amount of body fat. At first glance, pinching a fold of

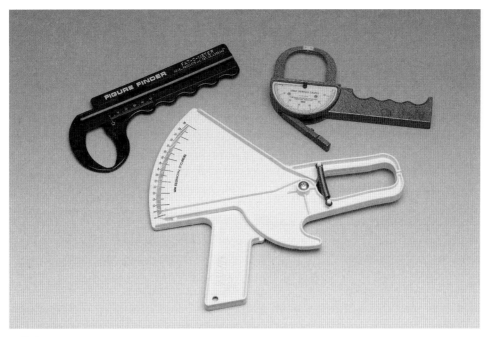

Figure 3.6 Range in quality of skinfold calipers.

skin and applying a set of calipers to measure the distance appears to be a simple skill. However, consistently obtaining accurate skinfold measurements requires a good-quality skinfold caliper, specific training, and a significant amount of practice, all of which are necessary to keep the potential error as small as possible.

The skinfold caliper should deliver a specific amount of force ($12 \text{ g} \cdot \text{mm}^{-2}$), and good-quality calipers come with this assurance from the manufacturer. Figure 3.6 provides examples of different types of skinfold calipers, which vary in quality. One source of variability in skinfold measurement occurs from using a caliper that does not deliver the recommended amount of force. Ideally, this level of force should be checked periodically; however, because most facilities lack the necessary instrumentation to do this, it is seldom done. The caliper distance measurement should also be checked using a simple standardized calibration block, as shown in Figure 3.7.

The skinfold procedure requires that the technician grasp the skin with the thumb and index finger ~3 in (7.5 cm) apart and firmly pull the skin, with the underlying subcutaneous fat, away from the limb

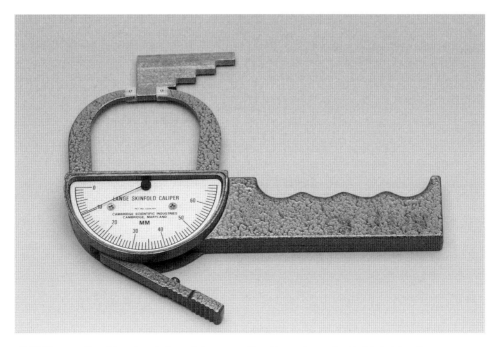

Figure 3.7 The method to check the distance calibration of a pair of skinfold calipers.

or torso. The fold will contain two layers of skin with only fat in between. If there is any doubt about the fold containing some muscle tissue, the client should be instructed to contract the muscle at that site to allow the technician to feel whether any muscle exists in the fold. The arms of the caliper are opened and applied to the skinfold by gradually releasing the pressure on the caliper arms. Note that the measurement scale should be facing up for viewing, which for most calipers requires a right-handed grip. Box 3.2 provides descriptions of the standardized skinfold sites along with procedural recommendations, as shown in Figure 3.8A–G. Careful attention to the anatomic landmarks and the actual measurement of distances is important for obtaining accurate and reliable measures. Once the location is identified, it should be marked on the skin with a water-solvent ink pen. Variation in the location of the skinfold site and the application of the calipers create the largest sources of error in skinfold measures. Figure 3.9A and B gives examples of correct and incorrect procedures for skinfold assessments, respectively.

As mentioned, the process of body fat estimation includes the calculation of Db and the conversion of Db to percent body fat. The most commonly used method for estimating Db via skinfold measurement employs the generalized equations provided in Box 3.3. For both men and women, there are three separate options to determine Db: one that uses seven skinfold sites and two that use three different skinfold sites (7,8). Theoretically, the more skinfold sites measured, the better the prediction of body fat. However, for most clients, there are minimal differences between the three- and seven-site methods, so the three-site methods are typically used. Because the proportion of subcutaneous to total fat is known to vary between sexes, between ethnic groups, and with age, different prediction equations have been developed to estimate body fat percentage. There are also generalized equations that can be used for most clients as well as specialized population-specific equations that can be used if working with a homogeneous group of people (*e.g.*, female collegiate volleyball players; Table 3.1).

Box 3.2   Standardized Description of Skinfold Sites and Procedures

Skinfold Site

Abdominal	Vertical fold; 2 cm to the right side of the umbilicus
Triceps	Vertical fold; on the posterior midline of the upper arm, halfway between the acromion and olecranon processes, with the arm held freely to the side of the body
Biceps	Vertical fold; on the anterior aspect of the arm over the belly of the biceps muscle, 1 cm above the level used to mark the triceps site
Chest/pectoral	Diagonal fold; one-half the distance between the anterior axillary line and the nipple (men), or one-third of the distance between the anterior axillary line and the nipple (women)
Medial calf	Vertical fold; at the maximum circumference of the calf on the midline of its medial border
Midaxillary	Vertical fold; on the midaxillary line at the level of the xiphoid process of the sternum. An alternate method is a horizontal fold taken at the level of the xiphoid/sternal border in the midaxillary line
Subscapular	Diagonal fold (at a 45-degree angle); 1–2 cm below the inferior angle of the scapula
Suprailiac	Diagonal fold; in line with the natural angle of the iliac crest taken in the anterior axillary line immediately superior to the iliac crest
Thigh	Vertical fold; on the anterior midline of the thigh, midway between the proximal border of the patella and the inguinal crease (hip)

Procedures
- All measurements should be made on the right side of the body with the subject standing upright.
- Caliper should be placed directly on the skin surface, 1 cm away from the thumb and finger, perpendicular to the skinfold, and halfway between the crest and the base of the fold.
- Pinch should be maintained while reading the caliper.
- Wait 1 to 2 s (not longer) before reading caliper.
- Take duplicate measures at each site and retest if duplicate measurements are not within 1 to 2 mm.
- Rotate through measurement sites or allow time for skin to regain normal texture and thickness.

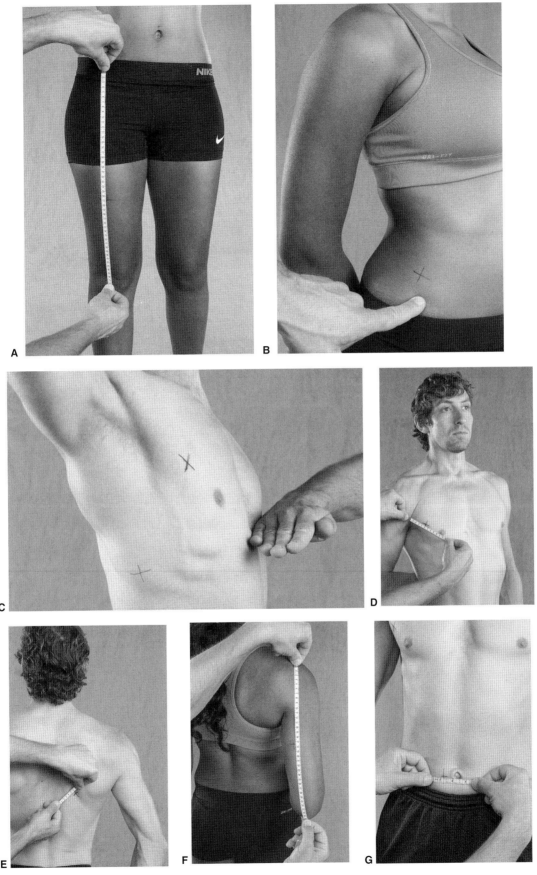

Figure 3.8 A: The thigh skinfold site. **B:** The suprailiac skinfold site. **C:** The midaxillary skinfold site. **D:** The chest skinfold site. **E:** The subscapular skinfold site. **F:** The triceps skinfold site. **G:** The abdomen skinfold site.

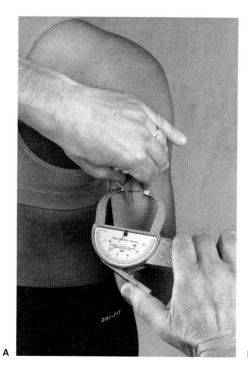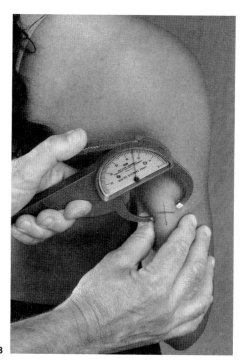

A
B

Figure 3.9 A: Example of the correct procedure for skinfold assessments. **B:** Example of an incorrect procedure for skinfold assessments.

Circumference Measurements

Circumference measurements have the advantages of being easily, inexpensively, and quickly administered, and the only equipment required is a measurement tape. Circumferences, also known as girths, are best used to measure changes in size of a body part. Perhaps the most important application is the

Box 3.3	Generalized Skinfold Equations

Men

- **Seven-Site Formula** (chest, midaxillary, triceps, subscapular, abdomen, suprailiac, and thigh)

    Body density = 1.112 − 0.00043499 (sum of seven skinfolds) + 0.00000055 (sum of seven skinfolds)^2 − 0.00028826 (age) *[SEE 0.008 or ~3.5% fat]*

- **Three-Site Formula** (chest, abdomen, and thigh)

    Body density = 1.10938 − 0.0008267 (sum of three skinfolds) + 0.0000016 (sum of three skinfolds)^2 − 0.0002574 (age) *[SEE 0.008 or ~3.4% fat]*

- **Three-Site Formula** (chest, triceps, and subscapular)

    Body density = 1.1125025 − 0.0013125 (sum of three skinfolds) + 0.0000055 (sum of three skinfolds)^2 − 0.000244 (age) *[SEE 0.008 or ~3.6% fat]*

Women

- **Seven-Site Formula** (chest, midaxillary, triceps, subscapular, abdomen, suprailiac, and thigh)

    Body density = 1.097 − 0.00046971 (sum of seven skinfolds) + 0.00000056 (sum of seven skinfolds)^2 − 0.00012828 (age) *[SEE 0.008 or ~3.8% fat]*

- **Three-Site Formula** (triceps, suprailiac, and thigh)

    Body density = 1.099421 − 0.0009929 (sum of three skinfolds) + 0.0000023 (sum of three skinfolds)^2 − 0.0001392 (age) *[SEE 0.009 or ~3.9% fat]*

- **Three-Site Formula** (triceps, suprailiac, and abdominal)

    Body density = 1.089733 − 0.0009245 (sum of three skinfolds) + 0.0000025 (sum of three skinfolds)^2 − 0.0000979 (age) *[SEE 0.009 or ~3.9% fat]*

SEE, standard error of estimate.
From Jackson AS, Pollock ML. Practical assessment of body composition. *Physician Sports Med.* 1985;13(5):76–90; Pollack M, Schmidt DH, Jackson A. Measurement of cardio-respiratory fitness and body composition in the clinical setting. *Compr Ther.* 1980;6(9):12–27.

use of circumferences to determine body fat distribution, as was covered in Chapter 2. Circumferences can also be used to measure muscle girth size and therefore quantify changes in muscle with specific training (*e.g.*, resistance weight training) or to help monitor sarcopenia. Training and/or age-related muscle change is most commonly measured in the limbs. For this purpose, measurement of the arm, forearm, midthigh, and calf are recommended.

Some equations estimating body fat percentages from circumference measurements are available for both sexes and a wide range of age groups (9–11). Box 3.4 provides descriptions of the standardized circumference sites along with procedural recommendations.

BIOELECTRICAL IMPEDANCE ANALYSIS

Yet another method for estimating body fat percentage, particularly popular in commercial fitness settings, is the bioelectrical impedance analysis (BIA). The bioelectrical impedance analyzer introduces a small electrical current into the body and measures the resistance to that current as it passes through the body. Current will flow more readily through water in the body, which contains electrolytes. Fat contains only small amounts of water so current will not flow as easily (*i.e.*, impeded) through areas containing fat. Conversely, lean tissue, which contains large amounts of water, and thus electrolytes, will be a good electrical conductor.

In general, BIA accuracy is similar to skinfold measurements as long as the protocol given below is being followed. Because the BIA measure is dependent on total body water and is based on assumptions about water content of fat and lean tissues, anything that changes a person's hydration status will affect the prediction of body fat percentage. Patients who are prescribed a medication that has a diuretic

Box 3.4	**Standardized Description of Circumference Sites and Procedures**
Abdomen	With the subject standing upright and relaxed, a horizontal measure is taken at the height of the iliac crest, usually at the level of the umbilicus.
Arm	With the subject standing erect and arms hanging freely at the sides with hands facing the thigh, a horizontal measure is taken midway between the acromion and olecranon processes.
Buttocks/hips	With the subject standing erect and feet together, a horizontal measure is taken at the maximal circumference of buttocks. This measure is used for the hip measure in a waist/hip measure.
Calf	With the subject standing erect (feet apart ~20 cm), a horizontal measure is taken at the level of the maximum circumference between the knee and the ankle, perpendicular to the long axis.
Forearm	With the subject standing, arms hanging downward but slightly away from the trunk and palms facing anteriorly, a measure is taken perpendicular to the long axis at the maximal circumference.
Hips/thigh	With the subject standing, legs slightly apart (~10 cm), a horizontal measure is taken at the maximal circumference of the hip/proximal thigh, just below the gluteal fold.
Midthigh	With the subject standing and one foot on a bench so the knee is flexed at 90 degrees, a measure is taken midway between the inguinal crease and the proximal border of the patella, perpendicular to the long axis.
Waist	With the subject standing, arms at the sides, feet together, and abdomen relaxed, a horizontal measure is taken at the narrowest part of the torso (above the umbilicus and below the xiphoid process). The National Obesity Task Force (NOTF) suggests obtaining a horizontal measure directly above the iliac crest as a method to enhance standardization. Unfortunately, current formulas are not predicated on the NOTF suggested site.

Procedures
- All measurements should be made with a flexible yet inelastic tape measure.
- The tape should be placed on the skin surface without compressing the subcutaneous adipose tissue.
- If a Gulick spring-loaded handle is used, the handle should be extended to the same marking with each trial.
- Take duplicate measures at each site and retest if duplicate measurements are not within 5 mm.
- Rotate through measurement sites or allow time for skin to regain normal texture.

Modified from Hales CM, Carroll MD, Fryar CD, Ogden CL. Prevalence of obesity among adults and youth: United States, 2015–2016. *NCHS Data Brief*. 2017;(288):1–8.

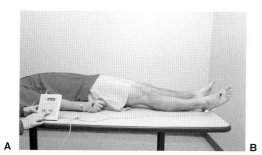
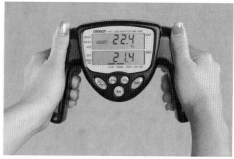

Figure 3.10 A: A bioelectrical impedance analysis (BIA) device that uses electrodes on the hand and foot. **B:** A handheld BIA device. Source: Photograph by Ball State University.

property should avoid this test because the results will probably not be valid. To control for factors that affect hydration status, the following pretest conditions should be used prior to a BIA measurement:

- No alcohol consumption for the previous 48 hours before the test
- No products with diuretic properties for the previous 24 hours before the test
- No exercise for the previous 12 hours before the test
- No eating or drinking for the previous 4 hours before the test
- Bladder should be voided completely within 30 minutes of the test

The procedures for BIA measurement are specific to the actual BIA device that is being used, and (see different BIA devises in Figure 3.10A and B) calibration of most devices is limited to an internal system check. Some devices require placing electrodes on the hand and foot to collect the necessary information, whereas others require a person to hold handles or stand on a platform to gather the information. There are no specific procedural requirements for the clients; yet, prior to the measurement, demographic data, including age, sex, height, and weight, are entered. Ideally, the client should have height and weight measured according to the procedures outlined in Chapter 2. A few of the BIA devices may also allow input of some category of physical activity status as well as ethnic/racial group. Similar to the skinfold method, BIA estimates of body fat percentage can be made from either generalized or population-specific equations, and some BIA devices allow the user to select an equation. Generally, most devices do not report the actual impedance values, so the raw data are unavailable for use in other equations.

INTERPRETATION

There are no universally accepted norms for body composition; however, the American College of Sports Medicine (ACSM) uses the reference values established by the Cooper Institute, as shown in Tables 3.2 and 3.3, for interpretation of body fat. It is important to recognize that these values are devised from only the population tested at the Cooper Institute, which represents a wide range of health conditions and ages, and there are known physiologic body composition changes associated with aging. For example, it is well accepted that bone mass and density decline with age, particularly in postmenopausal women. However, many of the changes observed in different age groups in adult populations regarding body fat percentage may actually be attributed to changes in lifestyle (physical activity and diet) rather than to the physiologic changes of aging. Thus, the 50th percentile of body fat according to Cooper data, although representing an average for a given population, does not necessarily represent a desirable value from a health and fitness standpoint. Based on skinfold reference values, the *ACSM's Guidelines for Exercise Testing and Prescription, Eleventh Edition (GETP11)* reports the "good" category range of 12% to 23% body fat for men and 17% to 26% body fat for women (12). However, there are limited data to support any true criterion-based approach for interpreting body fat results. Also as discussed in Chapter 1, whenever an assessment is based on estimation, the interpretation should include an expression of the standard error of the estimate (SEE). Table 3.4 provides the SEE values for hydrostatic weighing, plethysmography, skinfolds, and BIA.

TABLE 3.2 • Fitness Categories for Body Composition (% Body Fat) for Men by Age

Percentage		20–29	30–39	40–49	50–59	60–69	70–79
		Age (Years)					
99	Very lean[a]	4.2	7.3	9.5	11.0	11.9	13.6
95		6.4	10.3	12.9	14.8	16.2	15.5
90		7.9	12.4	15.0	17.0	18.1	17.5
85	Excellent	9.1	13.7	16.4	18.3	19.2	19.0
80		10.5	14.9	17.5	19.4	20.2	20.1
75		11.5	15.9	18.5	20.2	21.0	21.0
70	Good	12.6	16.8	19.3	21.0	21.7	21.6
65		13.8	17.7	20.1	21.7	22.4	22.3
60		14.8	18.4	20.8	22.3	23.0	22.9
55		15.8	19.2	21.4	23.0	23.6	23.7
50	Fair	16.6	20.0	22.1	23.6	24.2	24.1
45		17.5	20.7	22.8	24.2	24.9	24.7
40		18.6	21.6	23.5	24.9	25.6	25.3
35		19.7	22.4	24.2	25.6	26.4	25.8
30	Poor	20.7	23.2	24.9	26.3	27.0	26.5
25		22.0	24.1	25.7	27.1	27.9	27.1
20		23.3	25.1	26.6	28.1	28.8	28.4
15		24.9	26.4	27.8	29.2	29.8	29.4
10		26.6	27.8	29.2	30.6	31.2	30.7
5	Very poor	29.2	30.2	31.3	32.7	33.3	32.9
1		33.4	34.4	35.2	36.4	36.8	37.2
n =		1,844	10,099	15,073	9,255	2,851	522

Total n = 39,644

[a]Very lean, no less than 3% body fat is recommended for men.

Adapted with permission from Physical Fitness Assessments and Norms for Adults and Law Enforcement. The Cooper Institute, Dallas, Texas. 2009. For more information: www.cooperinstitute.org

TABLE 3.3 • Fitness Categories for Body Composition (% Body Fat) for Women by Age

Percentage		20–29	30–39	40–49	50–59	60–69	70–79
		Age (Years)					
99	Very lean[a]	11.4	11.2	12.1	13.9	13.9	11.7
95		14.0	13.9	15.2	16.9	17.7	16.4
90		15.1	15.5	16.8	19.1	20.2	18.3
85	Excellent	16.1	16.5	18.3	20.8	22.0	21.2
80		16.8	17.5	19.5	22.3	23.3	22.5
75		17.6	18.3	20.6	23.6	24.6	23.7
70	Good	18.4	19.2	21.7	24.8	25.7	24.8
65		19.0	20.1	22.7	25.8	26.7	25.7
60		19.8	21.0	23.7	26.7	27.5	26.6
55		20.6	22.0	24.6	27.6	28.3	27.6
50	Fair	21.5	22.8	25.5	28.4	29.2	28.2
45		22.2	23.7	26.4	29.3	30.1	28.9
40		23.4	24.8	27.5	30.1	30.8	30.5
35		24.2	25.8	28.4	30.8	31.5	31.0
30	Poor	25.5	26.9	29.5	31.8	32.6	31.9
25		26.7	28.1	30.7	32.9	33.3	32.9
20		28.2	29.6	31.9	33.9	34.4	34.0

(continued)

TABLE 3.3 • Fitness Categories for Body Composition (% Body Fat) for Women by Age (*continued*)

Percentage		Age (Years)					
		20–29	30–39	40–49	50–59	60–69	70–79
15		30.5	31.5	33.4	35.0	35.6	35.3
10		33.5	33.6	35.1	36.1	36.6	36.4
5	Very poor	36.6	36.2	37.1	37.6	38.2	38.1
1		38.6	39.0	39.1	39.8	40.3	40.2
n =		1,250	4,130	5,902	4,118	1,450	295

Total *n* = 17,145

[a]Very lean, no less than 10%–13% body fat is recommended for women.

Adapted with permission from Physical Fitness Assessments and Norms for Adults and Law Enforcement. The Cooper Institute, Dallas, Texas. 2009. For more information: www.cooperinstitute.org

TABLE 3.4 • Standard Error of Estimate for Different Body Fat Assessment Methods

Method for Estimating Body Fat Percentage	Standard Error of Estimate (%)
Air displacement (BOD POD)	±2.2 to ±3.7
Bioelectrical impedance analysis	±3.5 to ±5
Dual-energy X-ray absorptiometry	±1.8
Skinfold measurements	±3.5[a]
Underwater weighing	±2.5

[a]May vary with each equation.

Adapted from American College of Sports Medicine. *ACSM's Resource Manual for Guidelines for Exercise Testing and Prescription*. 6th ed. Philadelphia, PA: Wolters Kluwer Health Ltd; 2009:277.

ESTIMATION OF GOAL BODY WEIGHT

For those individuals who desire to alter body composition, it is helpful to provide them with an estimation of body weight at a goal body fat percentage. A simple method to derive an estimate of a goal body weight is based on the following equation:

$$\text{Goal body weight} = \frac{\text{Fat-free body}}{(1 - [\text{Goal body fat percentage} / 100])}$$

An example of the calculation of goal body weight for a man who weighs 200 lb with an estimated body fat of 25% and a goal body fat of 15% is as follows:

Determine fat-free weight:

$$\text{Fat-free body weight} = \text{Body weight} \times \left(\frac{[100 - \text{Body fat percentage}]}{100}\right)$$

$$= 200 \times \left(\frac{[100 - 25]}{100}\right) = 150 \text{ lb}$$

Determine goal body weight:

$$\text{Goal body weight} = \frac{150}{(1 - [15/100])} = 176.5 \text{ lb}$$

This approach uses the assumption that all of the weight that is lost is body fat.

SUMMARY

Body composition measurements are performed as part of a fitness evaluation and also provide important information related to functional status. Although there is no true gold standard measure of body composition, there are many methods that can provide helpful information.

LABORATORY ACTIVITIES

Skinfold Estimation of Body Fat Percentage

Data Collection

Work in groups of three and make all skinfold measurements on every member of your group (one technician, one subject, one recorder). Use Box 3.2 as a guide for identifying appropriate skinfold sites. Take each measurement twice (take a third if the first two differ by more than 2 mm) and average the two closest measures. Use Box 3.3 to calculate Db from skinfold measurements, and use the appropriation formula from Table 3.1 to calculate fat percentage from Db (when using Db to calculate body fat percentage, carry the Db value out four places past the decimal). Calculate your body fat using the seven-site formula and *each* of the three-site formulas in Box 3.3. Show your calculations on a separate sheet of paper and hand them in with the rest of the assignment. Record the values obtained on you.

Written Report

1. Using your fat percentage value for the seven-site formula for the first technician, what range of values would represent ±1 SEE unit encompassing 68% of the population with these same fat percentage values?
2. How did the fat percentage values obtained from the seven- and three-site formulas compare for the first technician?
3. How reliable were the two technicians in determining body fat percentage and the skinfold measures at each site?
4. Using the seven-site formula, what is your fat weight from each technician?
5. Using the seven-site formula, what is your fat-free weight from each technician?
6. Compare the body fat percentile with the classification of disease risk based on BMI and waist circumference (see Table 3.3). Are these two interpretations consistent?

Technician: _____ Height (in or cm): _____ Weight (lb or kg): _____

	Skinfolds			Mean
Abdominal	_____ mm	_____ mm	_____ mm	= _____ mm
Triceps	_____ mm	_____ mm	_____ mm	= _____ mm
Biceps	_____ mm	_____ mm	_____ mm	= _____ mm
Chest/pectoral	_____ mm	_____ mm	_____ mm	= _____ mm
Midaxillary	_____ mm	_____ mm	_____ mm	= _____ mm
Subscapular	_____ mm	_____ mm	_____ mm	= _____ mm
Suprailiac	_____ mm	_____ mm	_____ mm	= _____ mm
Thigh	_____ mm	_____ mm	_____ mm	= _____ mm

Seven-site formula: _____% fat

Three-site formula: _____% fat

Three-site formula: _____% fat

	Circumference			Mean
Waist	_____ cm	_____ cm	_____ cm	= cm

REFERENCES

1. Diemer EW, Grant JD, Munn-Chernoff MA, Patterson DA, Duncan AE. Gender identity, sexual orientation, and eating-related pathology in a national sample of college students. *J Adolesc Health*. 2015;57(2):144–9.
2. Trombetti A, Reid K, Hars M, et al. Age-associated declines in muscle mass, strength, power, and physical performance: impact on fear of falling and quality of life. *Osteoporos Int*. 2016;27(2):463–71.
3. Hales CM, Carroll MD, Fryar CD, Ogden CL. Prevalence of obesity among adults and youth: United States, 2015–2016. *NCHS Data Brief*. 2017;(288):1–8.
4. Walston JD. Sarcopenia in older adults. *Curr Opin Rheumatol*. 2012;24(6):623.
5. Boren HG, Kory RC, Syner JC. The Veterans Administration-Army cooperative study of pulmonary function: II. The lung volume and its subdivisions in normal men. *Am J Med*. 1966;41(1):96–114.
6. O'Brien RJ, Drizd TA. Roentgenographic determination of total lung capacity: normal values from a national population survey. *Am Rev Respir Dis*. 1983;128(5):949–52.
7. Jackson AS, Pollock ML. Practical assessment of body composition. *Phys Sportsmed*. 1985;13(5):76–90.
8. Pollack M, Schmidt DH, Jackson A. Measurement of cardio-respiratory fitness and body composition in the clinical setting. *Compr Ther*. 1980;6(9):12–27.
9. Tran ZV, Weltman A. Predicting body composition of men from girth measurements. *Hum Biol*. 1988;60:167–75.
10. Tran ZV, Weltman A. Generalized equation for predicting body density of women from girth measurements. *Med Sci Sports Exerc*. 1989;21(1):101–4.
11. Heyward VH, Wagner DR. *Applied Body Composition Assessment*. 2nd ed. Champaign: Human Kinetics; 2004.
12. ACSM. *ACSM's Guidelines for Exercise Testing and Prescription*. 11th ed. Wolters Kluwer; 2021.

Estimation of Cardiorespiratory Fitness from Field and Submaximal Exercise Tests

WHY MEASURE CARDIORESPIRATORY FITNESS

Cardiorespiratory fitness (CRF) reflects the functional capabilities of the heart, blood vessels, lungs, and skeletal muscles to perform work. As such, CRF is often considered one of the best indicators of the collective health and function of the entire body and a vital sign for cardiovascular health (1). CRF provides the ability to perform large muscle, dynamic, moderate- to high-intensity exercise for prolonged periods. There are many different terms that have been used to describe this measure of physical fitness, including the following:

- Maximal aerobic capacity
- Functional capacity
- Physical work capacity
- Cardiovascular endurance, fitness, or capacity
- Cardiorespiratory endurance, fitness, or capacity
- Cardiopulmonary endurance, fitness, or capacity

There are a multitude of desirable outcomes that can be derived from the assessment of CRF. Some of these outcomes are derived from additional measurements (*e.g.*, an electrocardiogram [ECG]) that are recorded during the exercise test when determining CRF. Purely from a fitness perspective, CRF can be used to provide motivation for a participant considering participation in a physical activity/exercise program, to individualize the exercise prescription, and to track progress within an exercise program.

Another important value of the assessment of CRF is that it directly relates to a participant's functional status, as noted by the use of the term *functional capacity* to describe CRF. This can be demonstrated, in part, by comparing a 45-year-old woman with high (85th percentile) CRF (11.4 metabolic equivalents [METs]) to one with low (15th percentile) CRF (7.6 METs). The woman with high CRF can easily perform occupational and recreational activities that require 6 to 9 METs, such as carrying groceries upstairs, riding a bicycle at 10 mph, shoveling snow, or playing singles tennis (2). The woman with low CRF will only be able to perform these same activities, if at all, with maximal or near-maximal effort and will fatigue quickly. Two other functional reasons for assessing CRF involve clinical decisions regarding work. First, CRF results can aid in making occupational disability determinations and can also provide a component of a return-to-work evaluation for participants with an occupation that involves regular aerobic activity. Second, CRF, in combination with other exercise test measurements, can provide valuable clinical information, both prognostic and diagnostic, for patients with or without chronic diseases (3). Furthermore, considerable evidence exists to clearly demonstrate the importance of CRF both as a prognostic tool in apparently healthy men and women (1) and as a superior predictor of mortality when compared to tobacco use, hypertension, elevated lipids, and diabetes mellitus (4). Lastly, modest improvements in CRF (~1 MET) provide significant improvements in overall survival (1).

The American College of Sports Medicine (ACSM) Guidelines for Exercise Testing and Prescription, Eleventh Edition (GETP11) contains an abstract of the clinical use of the exercise test (see Chapter 4) and summarizes the evidence that establishes a low level of CRF as an independent risk factor for all-cause and cardiovascular mortality.

WHAT IS THE GOLD STANDARD MEASURE OF CARDIORESPIRATORY FITNESS?

The gold standard measure of CRF is the maximal exercise test with collection of expired gases. This test is performed in a laboratory setting, with trained personnel, and requires specific monitoring equipment as discussed in Chapter 5. Because this method involves time, cost, and skilled personnel, as well as a higher level of risk, it is not always feasible or desired. It should be noted that maximal exercise testing is also performed in clinical settings for diagnosis and prognosis of some chronic diseases. Fortunately, there are many alternative approaches that provide estimates of CRF using submaximal protocols following established field or laboratory tests.

FIELD TESTS FOR PREDICTION OF CARDIORESPIRATORY FITNESS

Field tests occur in various nonlaboratory settings (*i.e.*, in the "field") and are typically administered to a group of people simultaneously. Most commonly, these tests require participants to (a) complete a certain distance as quickly as possible, (b) cover as much distance as possible in a fixed amount of time, or (c) perform a set amount of work in a fixed amount of time. Field tests can be either maximal or submaximal in effort.

Many field tests originated from the need to assess CRF of a large group in a time-efficient, non-laboratory setting. Field tests have several advantages over lab tests: they do not require highly trained personnel to administer them, they are time-efficient, many participants are tested in one session, and they are inexpensive, requiring little, if any, equipment. Generally, these types of tests are considered safe to perform; however, this may be because they are typically used in younger, low-risk populations. It is important to recognize that some of the tests, such as running 1.5 mi as fast as possible, will result in a maximal or near-maximal level of exertion. This requirement may be inappropriate for participants at moderate-to-high risk for cardiovascular or musculoskeletal complications. Performing the screening procedures, as reviewed in Chapter 2, on all participants prior to a CRF assessment and following the personnel recommendations for supervision are thus warranted.

Step Tests

Step test protocols that include a fixed stepping rate and step height tend to produce less accurate CRF values compared to protocols individualized for stepping rate and stature, as the required cadence and step height may be inappropriate for the participant (5). Moreover, the results are easy to explain to the participant after the test is completed (6). These tests are typically performed with younger populations; therefore, precautions should be considered for those with balance problems or those who are extremely deconditioned. For example, some single-stage step tests require an energy cost of 7 to 9 METs, which may exceed the maximal capacity of some participants (7). Therefore, the protocol chosen must be appropriate for the physical fitness level of the participant. Once chosen, it is important that all test procedures (*i.e.*, step height, cadence) are followed, as this impacts the accuracy of the test. Table 5.3 provides a summary of common step test protocols.

The original Harvard two-step test was first used in medicine to aid in the diagnosis of heart disease (8). Many alternative methods have been developed since; however, most involve a participant performing a fixed amount of work in a set amount of time, followed by the measurement of heart rate (HR) response. The McArdle or Queens College step test is often used to simultaneously assess large groups of participants to predict their CRF (9). The procedures for the Queens College step test are provided in Box 4.1. Note that any changes to the procedure, including using a different step height or a different rate of stepping, will invalidate the results.

In addition to the Queens College step test, several other multistage step tests are also possible (Table 4.1). For example, the Webb protocol, designed for college-aged adults, increases stepping

---

Box 4.1   Queens College Step Test Procedures

1. The step test requires that the participant step up and down on a standardized step height of 16.25 in (41.25 cm) for 3 minutes. (Many gymnasium bleachers have a riser height of 16.25 in.)
2. Men step at a rate (cadence) of 24 per minute, whereas women step at a rate of 22 per minute. This cadence should be closely monitored and set with the use of an electronic metronome. A 24-step-per-minute cadence means that the complete cycle of step up with one leg, step up with the other, step down with the first leg, and finally step down with the last leg is performed 24 times in a minute. Commonly, the metronome is set at a cadence of four times the step rate, in this case 96 bpm for men, to coordinate each leg's movement with a beat of the metronome. The women's step cadence would be 88 bpm. Although it may be possible to test more than one participant at a time, the group would need to be of the same gender.
3. At the conclusion of 3 minutes, the participant stops and palpates the pulse (typically at the radial site) while standing, within the first 5 seconds. A 15-second pulse count is then taken and multiplied by four to determine the HR in bpm. This recovery HR should occur within the first 30 seconds of immediate recovery from the end of the step test. The subject's $\dot{V}O_{2max}$ is determined from the recovery HR by the following formulas:

$$\text{For men: } \dot{V}O_{2max} \text{ (mL} \cdot \text{kg}^{-1} \cdot \text{min}^{-1}) = 111.33 - (0.42 \times HR)$$
$$\text{For women: } \dot{V}O_{2max} \text{ (mL} \cdot \text{kg}^{-1} \cdot \text{min}^{-1}) = 65.81 - (0.1847 \times HR)$$

For example, if a man finished the test with a recovery HR = 144 bpm (36 beats in 15 s), then

$$\dot{V}O_{2max} \text{ (mL} \cdot \text{kg}^{-1} \cdot \text{min}^{-1}) = 111.33 - (0.42 \times 144)$$
$$= 50.85 \text{ mL} \cdot \text{kg}^{-1} \cdot \text{min}^{-1}$$

The Queens College step test is also known as the McArdle step test (10).

TABLE 4.1 • Summary of Common Step Tests				
Test	Population	Step Height (cm)	Step Rate (steps · min⁻¹)	Duration
Åstrand-Ryhming (7)	Healthy adults	Women: 33 Men: 40	22.5	5 min
Webb (11)	Young adults	Individualized (0.19 × stature in cm)	Variable; dependent on perceived functional ability; increased by 5 steps · min⁻¹ every 2 min	75% of age-predicted HR_{max}
YMCA (10)	Healthy adults	30.5	24	3 min
Queens College (9)	Young adults	41.3	Women: 22 Men: 24	3 min
STEP Tool (12)	All adults	20	Variable	20 stepping cycles

HR_{max}, maximal heart rate.

cadence by 5 steps · min⁻¹ every 2 minutes until 75% of the age-predicted HR_{max} (APMHR) is attained (11). For this test, step height is individualized based on the participant's height. To estimate maximal volume of oxygen consumed per unit time ($\dot{V}O_{2max}$), the final stepping cadence, the recovery HR at 45 seconds, and the individualized perceived functional ability are needed. Such step tests should be modified to suit the population being tested.

In addition, the 3-minute YMCA step test uses a 12-in (30.5-cm) bench, with a stepping rate of 24 steps · min⁻¹ (estimated $\dot{V}O_2$ of 25.8 mL · kg⁻¹ · min⁻¹). After stepping is completed, the subject immediately sits down, and HR is counted for 1 minute. Counting must start within 5 seconds at the end of exercise. HR values are used to obtain a qualitative rating of fitness from published normative tables (10).

Fixed Distance Tests

There are two common field test protocols that predict CRF by using a walk or run performance of a fixed distance. The performance tests can be classified into walk/run tests, where the participant walks or runs or uses a combination of both to complete the test, or a pure walk test, where the participant is strictly limited to walking the entire test. The 1-mile (mi) walk test is generally indicated for those who have been sedentary or irregularly active or are unable to run because of an injury. The participant should be able to walk briskly for 1 mi to be a good candidate for this test.

Prior to any test, it is important to inform the participant of the purpose of the test (*i.e.*, to estimate CRF) and to emphasize that it is critical to find the best pace to cover the specific distance in the shortest amount of time possible. Effective pacing and subject motivation are key determinants in the outcome of this test. For many people, especially those who do not exercise regularly, finding the ideal pace takes practice. Thus, because a learning effect is likely for most people, it is ideal to perform these tests more than once on different days to obtain an accurate estimate of CRF.

The 1-mi walk test requires the participant to walk 1 mi as quickly as possible around a measured course. *Walking* is defined as having one foot in contact with the ground at all times (running involves an airborne phase). The test requires an accurate measure of body weight prior to the test, a clock to time the duration of the walk, and the ability to measure the participant's HR at the completion of the walk. The HR measured at the completion of the walk is considered the "peak" HR. The use of an HR monitor is preferred; however, a 15-second pulse count can be used if needed. Immediately following the 1-mi walk, the time to complete the test and the HR at the end of the test are recorded. If pulse palpation is used, the participant counts the recovery pulse for 15 seconds and multiplies by 4 to determine the peak HR (beats per minute [bpm]). It is important to begin the pulse count within 5 seconds of test completion, and the subject should keep the legs moving to prevent pooling of blood in the periphery, which could lead to light-headedness. The formula to calculate estimated CRF is provided in Box 4.2 (13).

The 1.5-mi run test requires the participant to complete this distance in the shortest time possible either by running the whole distance or by combining running with periods of walking. Ideally, the

Box 4.2   Prediction of Cardiorespiratory Fitness from the 1-mi Walk Test

$$\dot{V}O_{2max} \text{ (mL} \cdot \text{kg}^{-1} \cdot \text{min}^{-1}) = 132.853 - (0.1692 \times wt) - (0.3877 \times age) + (6.315 \times sex) - (3.2649 \times time) - (0.1565 \times HR)$$

where
  wt = weight in kilograms
  age = in years
  sex = 0 (women) or 1 (men)
  time = min (remember to convert seconds to minutes by dividing by 60) (*e.g.*, [42/60 = 0.7])
  HR = recovery heart rate in bpm

EXAMPLE

A 32-year-old man who weighed 170 lb completed the test in 12 minutes and 36 seconds with a 15-second pulse count of 35 bpm.

Conversions:

$$\text{Weight pounds to kilograms: } 170/2.2 = 77.3 \text{ kg}$$
$$\text{Time to minutes: } 12 + (36/60) = 12.6 \text{ min}$$
$$\text{Pulse in 15 seconds to HR: } 35 \times 4 = 140 \text{ bpm}$$
$$\dot{V}O_{2max} \text{ (mL} \cdot \text{kg}^{-1} \cdot \text{min}^{-1}) = 132.853 - (0.1692 \times 77.3) - (0.3877 \times 32) + (6.315 \times 1) - (3.2649 \times 12.6) - (0.1565 \times 140)$$
$$\dot{V}O_{2max} \text{ (mL} \cdot \text{kg}^{-1} \cdot \text{min}^{-1}) = 50.6 \text{ mL} \cdot \text{kg}^{-1} \cdot \text{min}^{-1}$$

This formula was derived from apparently healthy participants ranging in age from 30 to 69 years (13).

participant should be able to jog for 15 minutes continuously to obtain a reasonable prediction of CRF. This test is best performed on a track and requires only a stopwatch/clock to administer. Once the test is completed, $\dot{V}O_{2max}$ can be estimated based on the amount of time it took the participant to complete the specified distance using the following formula:

$$\dot{V}O_{2max} \text{ (mL} \cdot \text{kg}^{-1} \cdot \text{min}^{-1}) = 3.5 + 483/1.5 \text{ mi time (min)}$$

Fixed Time Tests

Another variation of the 1.5-mi run test is the 12-minute walk/run test popularized by Dr. Ken Cooper of the Cooper Aerobics Clinic in Dallas, Texas. This test requires the participant to cover the maximum possible distance in 12 minutes by walking or running or using a combination of both. The distance covered in 12 minutes needs to be measured and expressed in meters. Once the test is complete, CRF can be estimated using the following equation:

$$\dot{V}O_{2max} \text{ (mL} \cdot \text{kg}^{-1} \cdot \text{min}^{-1}) = (\text{distance in meters} - 504.9)/44.73$$

In clinical populations who are very deconditioned, the 6-minute walk test is a common fixed distance test that is used to estimate CRF. In addition, this test is used as an outcome measure to evaluate progress in rehabilitation programs, and although it is considered a good indicator of functional capacity in deconditioned patients, it has generally not been a good predictor of measured $\dot{V}O_{2max}$ (14).

SUBMAXIMAL EXERCISE TESTS FOR PREDICTION OF CARDIORESPIRATORY FITNESS

A submaximal exercise test is one that requires the participant to perform a fixed amount of work per unit of time, and in many cases, these tests require multiple stages or levels. The key distinguishing feature of these tests is that they limit the participant's effort to less than maximal exertion. There are several protocols that may be used to conduct submaximal exercise tests to predict CRF using various testing modalities, from the bench step, to the cycle ergometer, to the treadmill. Although some versions of step tests are done in a medical/fitness setting, this form of administration is much less common than the use of the test within a field setting. Submaximal tests require participants to exercise on a particular mode (*e.g.*, treadmill, cycle ergometer) at a known work output that is less than their maximal effort.

Throughout the test, the participant's HR should be measured at different work outputs, and this information is used to estimate CRF. Overall, the cycle ergometer provides a more exact quantification of work than other comparable exercise testing modes, such as the treadmill. This accuracy provides a better ability to calculate the exact work output that is important when trying to estimate CRF.

Assumptions for Submaximal Exercise Tests

The prediction of CRF from submaximal tests will have some error; thus, certain assumptions must be made. These assumptions include the following:

- Between a HR of 110 and 150 bpm, everyone has a linear (straight line) relationship between $\dot{V}O_2$ and HR. This is a fairly robust assumption, meaning that it is largely true. In exercise physiology, we know that once the stroke volume has reached a "plateau" (around 40%–50% of max), the HR and $\dot{V}O_2$ track linearly (15).
- HR_{max}, which must be predicted for submaximal ergometer testing, can be estimated or predicted because it is a function of age. Unfortunately, there is a large standard deviation for the age prediction of HR_{max}, and this assumption may provide for the greatest error in submaximal ergometer prediction of CRF.
- Steady-state heart rate (HRss) — a steady physiologic response can be achieved in 3 to 4 minutes at a constant, submaximal work output. This is a largely achievable assumption by ensuring that a participant reaches a HRss during each and every stage of the protocol chosen. Thus, the achievement of HRss during the protocol is a very important concept and goal during any submaximal prediction of CRF test.
- The cadence of 50 revolutions per minute (rpm) is comfortable, and almost everybody is mechanically efficient at a 50 rpm cadence, although some may not be comfortable at this cadence. Everyone expends the same amount of energy and has the same absolute oxygen requirements at the same work output on the cycle. This assumption is the basis for ACSM's metabolic calculations (see Chapter 6).
- Submaximal work output can predict maximal work output and thus maximal aerobic capacity. This assumption is a part of the next assumption.
- The HR at two separate work outputs can be plotted as the HR-$\dot{V}O_2$ relationship and extrapolated to the estimated HR_{max}. Both the YMCA submaximal cycle ergometer protocol and the Bruce submaximal treadmill protocol are multistage tests that use the concept of at least two stages to predict CRF. The Åstrand protocol is only a single-stage test; this assumption does not directly apply to it.

In addition to multiple assumptions, submaximal exercise tests have several sources of error that will impact the prediction of CRF. These sources of error include the following:

1. Prediction of HR_{max} by age.
2. Efficiency of the participant performing the test in ergometer (*e.g.*, cycling).
3. Equipment calibration. Although sometimes taken for granted, calibration is vital to the accuracy of the test results.
4. Accurate measurement of HR during each stage.
5. Having an HRss at each stage.

Deciding on Which Method to Use

Even though the preferred method to evaluate CRF is a maximal effort test, the fitness professional should consider the status of the individuals prior to determining what type of test to complete. The most appropriate assessment to evaluate CRF is one that provides the most information while keeping the participant safe. Although a variety of assessments exist, factors that should be taken into account before deciding what method to use include the following:

- Reasons for the test
- Risk level
- Expense
- Time required
- Personnel required
- Equipment and facilities required

Box 4.3 **Advantages and Disadvantages of Submaximal Exercise Testing**

ADVANTAGES

- Relatively inexpensive and requires less equipment, personnel, and medical supervision than do maximal exercise tests
- Allows for testing of large groups
- Generally shorter test duration time
- If multistage test: can assess multiple HR and BP responses to standardized work outputs

DISADVANTAGES

- Maximal measurements (HR, BP, $\dot{V}O_2$) are not taken, but often predicted
- $\dot{V}O_{2max}$ prediction error can range around 10% to 20%
- Limited diagnostic utility for certain diseases, such as coronary heart disease
- Limited for exercise prescription purposes, with no measured HR_{max}

Because the alternatives to maximal lab testing involve the prediction of CRF, the estimation of error (standard error of estimate [SEE]), as discussed in Chapter 1, should be part of the decision process. When deciding if submaximal exercise testing is most appropriate to estimate CRF, the fitness professional should consider its advantages and disadvantages (Box 4.3).

PRETEST STANDARDIZATIONS FOR CARDIORESPIRATORY FITNESS ASSESSMENTS

To obtain optimal results, pretest instructions for participants to follow prior to performing a CRF assessment test should be provided. Participants should be instructed to wear comfortable exercise-type clothing, avoid tobacco and caffeine 3 hours prior to the test, avoid alcohol 12 hours prior to the test, consume plenty of fluids, avoid strenuous exercise for 24 hours prior to the test, and obtain an adequate amount of sleep the night before the test.

Prior to beginning any assessment, it is important that the participant has provided informed consent and, at a minimum, a PAR-Q has been provided as a screening tool. Performance instructions specific to the test should be reviewed with the participant. It is crucial that the participant understands that he or she is free to terminate the test at any time and is also responsible for informing the test administrator of any and all symptoms (*e.g.*, chest discomfort, fatigue) as they develop. In addition, an explanation of the rating of perceived exertion (RPE) scale is warranted at this time, if it is being used during the test. This scale, developed by Gunnar Borg, is provided in table 3.6 of *ACSM's GETP11*. Verbal directions should be read to the participant prior to the test for obtaining the RPE measurement. These directions should be consistent with the recommendations of Borg (16). A summary or general procedures for submaximal testing of CRF is provided in Box 4.4.

PREDICTING MAXIMAL HEART RATE

A fundamental feature of many submaximal exercise tests is the reliance on knowing the participant's HR_{max}. The measurement of HR_{max} requires a maximal exercise effort; thus, it cannot be obtained during submaximal exercise tests. Therefore, these submaximal testing procedures depend on the use of a prediction of HR_{max}, typically estimated from age. Although there are many different prediction equations for HR_{max} (see table 4.3 of *ACSM's GETP11*), many have large error estimate (SEE) ranging between 10 and 15 bpm. The most commonly used equation to predict age predicted HRmax is:

$$\text{Age-predicted } HR_{max} = 220 - \text{age (yr)}$$

However, this equation was developed "arbitrarily" from only a few studies and lacks utility for older adults (17). In 2001, Tanaka and colleagues (18) conducted a meta-analysis including 18,712 participants and confirmed the strong inverse relationship between age and HR_{max}, reporting an *r* value of −0.90 and yielding the following equation:

$$\text{Age-predicted } HR_{max} = 208 - 0.7 \text{ (age)}$$

Box 4.4	General Procedures for Submaximal Testing of Cardiorespiratory Fitness

1. Obtain resting HR and BP immediately prior to exercise in the exercise posture.
2. The participant should be familiarized with the ergometer. If using a cycle ergometer, properly position the participant on the ergometer (*i.e.*, upright posture, ~25-degree bend in the knee at maximal leg extension, and hands in proper position on handlebars) (15–17).
3. The exercise test should begin with a 2- to 3-minute warm-up to acquaint the participant with the cycle ergometer and prepare him or her for the exercise intensity in stage 1 of the test.
4. A specific protocol should consist of 2- or 3-minute stages with appropriate increments in work rate.
5. HR should be monitored at least two times during each stage, near the end of minute 2 and 3 of each stage. If HR is >110 bpm, HRss (*i.e.*, two HRs within 5 bpm) should be reached before the workload is increased.
6. BP should be monitored in the last minute of each stage and repeated (verified) in the event of a hypotensive or hypertensive response.
7. RPE (using either the Borg category or category-ratio scale; see table 4.6 from *GETP11*) and additional rating scales should be monitored near the end of the last minute of each stage.
8. Participant's appearance and symptoms should be monitored and recorded regularly.
9. The test should be terminated when the subject reaches 70% HRR (85% of APMHR), fails to conform to the exercise test protocol, experiences adverse signs or symptoms, requests to stop, or experiences an emergency situation.
10. An appropriate cool-down/recovery period should be initiated consisting of either
    a. continued exercise at a work rate equivalent to that of stage 1 of the exercise test protocol or lower or
    b. a passive cool-down if the subject experiences signs of discomfort or an emergency situation occurs.
11. All physiologic observations (*e.g.*, HR, BP, signs, and symptoms) should be continued for at least 5 minutes of recovery unless abnormal responses occur, which would warrant a longer posttest surveillance period. Continue low-level exercise until HR and BP stabilize, but not necessarily until they reach preexercise levels.

Even though some variability exists when estimating HR_{max}, these prediction equations work well for large groups. For example, if the HR_{max} of 100 40-year-olds were measured, the average HR_{max} for the group would be very close to 180 bpm. However, approximately one in three people in this group will have a true HR_{max} of either <165 bpm or >195 bpm. This large variability in APMHR is one of the sources of error in predicting CRF from submaximal exercise tests. Some actual measured HR_{max} at different ages are shown in Figure 4.1 (18).

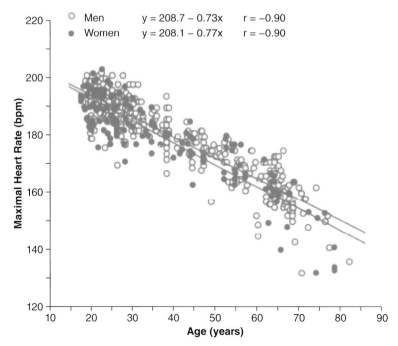

Figure 4.1 Variability in maximal heart rate at different ages between men and women. Source: Reprinted from reference [17], fig 1. Variability in maximal heart rate at different ages between men and women. Reprinted from Tanaka H, Monahan KD, Seals DR. Age-predicted maximal heart rate revisited. *J Am Coll Cardiol.* 2001;37(1):153–156. doi:10.1016/s0735-1097(00)01054-8.

Box 4.5   General Indications for Stopping an Exercise Test[a]

- Onset of angina or angina-like symptoms
- Drop in systolic blood pressure (SBP) of ≥10 mm Hg with an increase in work rate or if SBP decreases below the value obtained in the same position prior to testing
- Excessive rise in BP: SBP >250 mm Hg and/or diastolic BP >115 mm Hg
- Shortness of breath, wheezing, leg cramps, or claudication
- Signs of poor perfusion: light-headedness, confusion, ataxia, pallor, cyanosis, nausea, or cold and clammy skin
- Failure of HR to increase with increased exercise intensity
- Noticeable change in heart rhythm by palpation or auscultation
- Subject requests to stop
- Physical or verbal manifestations of severe fatigue
- Failure of the testing equipment

[a]Assumes that testing is nondiagnostic and is being performed without direct physician involvement or ECG monitoring. For clinical testing, the reader is referred to Chapter 4 of ACSM's GETP11.

LABORATORY MEASURES

Test Termination Criteria

Prior to the onset of a submaximal exercise test, clear exercise test endpoints should be established. One recommendation is to use a test termination criterion of 70% HR reserve (HRR) or 85% APMHR. This method should result in a submaximal effort for most participants. However, considering the variability of HR_{max} prediction equations, it needs to be understood that some participants will reach their actual HR_{max}. Thus, observing signs and symptoms of maximal effort may warrant termination of the test prior to attaining the test termination criteria of 70% HRR or 85% APMHR. ACSM has developed a list of general indications for stopping an exercise test in adults, which should be kept in mind when carrying out submaximal exercise tests (Box 4.5). As noted at the bottom of Box 4.5, there are other test termination criteria used in clinical exercise testing. These criteria for stopping an exercise test may need to be applied if the participant is at high risk for cardiovascular disease.

Monitoring

As with field tests, during any laboratory test, it is important to observe the participant for signs of distress and inquire about symptoms that would indicate test termination. For the actual assessment of CRF, HR monitoring is required, and this can be accomplished either with pulse palpation or with monitoring HR monitor. Because these tests are typically performed in a laboratory setting, adding blood pressure (BP) monitoring is sometimes desired. However, measuring BP during exercise involves a higher skill requirement for the technician. Note that BP monitoring is not used to estimate CRF; rather, it is an optional health risk assessment to evaluate a participant's BP response to exercise.

EXERCISE MODES

The most commonly used mode of exercise for submaximal exercise testing is the cycle ergometer. However, any exercise mode that allows for standardization of the work rates with known estimates of volume of oxygen consumed per unit time ($mL \cdot kg^{-1} \cdot min^{-1}$) can be used.

Cycle Ergometer

Even though cycle ergometers are most commonly used for submaximal testing, there are certain disadvantages that merit consideration. Most significant is that cycling is not a common mode of exercise or activity for many adults in the United States. In addition, mechanically braked cycle ergometers require the participant to maintain a constant pedaling cadence to keep the work rate constant. These

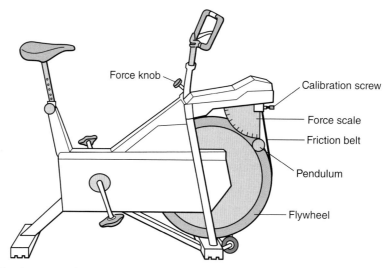

Figure 4.2 The features of a mechanically braked cycle ergometer. Source: Reprinted from Adams GM, Beam WC. *Exercise Physiology Laboratory Manual.* New York (NY): McGraw Hill; 2008. p. 137.

two factors may cause fatigue before reaching any meaningful endpoint, especially among older adults, minimizing the utility of the estimation.

Nonetheless, there are many more advantages to using a cycle ergometer that make it the primary mode of choice for submaximal exercise testing. First, the cycle ergometer is non–weight bearing, which makes it a good choice for participants with orthopedic limitations. Second, the cycle ergometer is a relatively safe mode of exercise, limiting the participants' risk of falling off the equipment — compared to a treadmill or even a step. Third, BP and pulse by palpation are more easily measured during exercise on the cycle ergometer because of the limited noise that the cycle produces as well as the natural stabilization of the upper body and arm. Lastly, cycle ergometers are less expensive and more portable than treadmills, require little space, and most have no electrical needs.

Currently, the mechanically braked Monark cycle ergometer is the most popular brand used for submaximal exercise testing because of the ease in calibrating the ergometer. An example of a mechanically braked cycle ergometer is shown in Figure 4.2. Calibration of this ergometer ensures accurate work outputs for the different stages of a submaximal test. The calibration procedure for the Monark cycle ergometer is provided in Box 4.6.

Box 4.6 Calibration of the Monark Cycle Ergometer

The calibration of the cycle ergometer is the first step and a very important step before performing a laboratory submaximal cycle exercise test. Prior to calibrating, examine the resistance belt and flywheel for excessive wear and dirt. For the Monark cycle static calibration (treadmill calibration is not covered in this manual as it varies between treadmill model),

1. Zero the ergometer by unfastening the resistance belt from the pendulum. (Note: The ergometer should be on a level surface.)
2. Examine the resistance belt and flywheel for excessive wear and dirt — both the belt and the flywheel should be clean. The flywheel can be cleaned with steel wool and cleanser, and the belt can also be cleaned with a mild detergent; however, you should not conduct a test if either is wet, so plan ahead. Most resistance belts have a life span of several years before they need replacing depending on usage.
3. Check to see that the resistance scale (on the side of the cycle) reads zero; if not, adjust to zero with the thumbscrew.
4. You may add a known weight to the shorter belt (*e.g.,* 1 kg) and check the resistance scale output to ensure that the resistance scale reads that weight (*e.g.,* 1 kg). It is better to attach a heavier calibration weight to magnify any potential error.
5. Finally, reattach the belt to the mechanism and be sure to pull the belt somewhat tight without too much slack. If you allow for too much slack in the belt when you reattach the belt, then the resistance mechanism may fail to provide you with the necessary resistance output range (*i.e.,* you will not be able to turn the resistance up to 3 kp or more). Likewise, if you pull the belt too tight, the cycle will not be able to be freewheeled. Check the Monark ergometer handbook to learn more about calibration of the cycle.

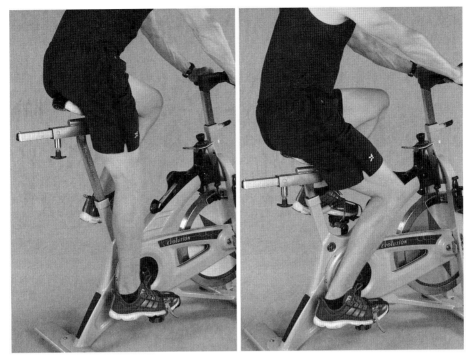

Figure 4.3 An example of a seat height set correctly (*left*) and too low (*right*) for cycle ergometer testing.

When using cycle ergometers, adequate calibration, along with proper seat height, is important for optimal performance; an incorrect setting can result in inefficiency and early fatigue. To maximize force production and leg muscle activation, the knee should be slightly bent when the sole of the foot is centered over the pedal axle with the pedal in the bottom position. Figure 4.3 illustrates a correct and an incorrect seat height setting. Proper positioning can be achieved in several ways. One, with the participant seated and the forefoot on the pedals, ask the participant to extend the leg to the pedal-down position. Adjust seat height based on comfort. Another way to check seat height is to have the participant place the heels on the pedals and with the foot in a dorsiflexed position ensure the leg is straight in the pedal-down position. Lastly, with the participant standing next to the cycle ergometer, align the seat with the participant's greater trochanter, or hip. Most importantly, the participant should actually sit on the bike, turn the pedals, and evaluate comfort with the seat height. While pedaling, the participant should feel comfortable, and there should be no rocking of the hips. In addition, the participant should maintain an upright posture, which may require an adjustment to the handlebars, and should not grip the handlebars too tightly.

Work Output Determination

Chapter 6 provides a more detailed description of the metabolic equations, which includes information on work output settings. As noted in Chapter 6, work is determined by multiplying force and distance. At times, resistance is presented as kilopond (kp), from Latin in which pondus means weight. Through this book, however, we use resistance as kilogram-force (kg). Work output, or power, is expressed in terms of how much work is performed per unit of time using the following equation:

$$\text{Work output } (\text{kg} \cdot \text{m}^{-1} \cdot \text{min}^{-1}) = \text{resistance} \times \text{cadence} \times \text{distance}$$

Resistance in this equation refers to the resistance caused on the flywheel by the pendulum weight and friction on the belt. This resistance is measured as a gravitational force in kilopond (kp) or as kilogram-force (kg). The kp (or kg) is the force exerted by the Earth's gravity by the swinging pendulum weight, applied to the friction belt on the flywheel of the cycle ergometer. Resistance can be increased during the test to apply standardized work outputs.

Cadence is simply the number of pedal rpm. Most common submaximal cycle protocols require a constant rate of 50 rpm. Newer ergometers usually have an electronic console that measures rpm; otherwise, the pedaling rate needs to be in cadence with a metronome set at 100 rpm (for 100 downstrokes

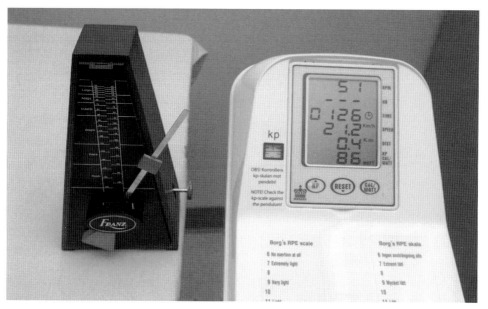

Figure 4.4 The use of a metronome to check the calibration of the revolutions per minute (rpm) meter on a cycle. Source: Photograph by Ball State University.

to produce 50 rpm). It is prudent to periodically verify that the console measure is reading accurately by cross-checking it with a metronome, as shown in Figure 4.4.

Distance here refers to the distance the flywheel travels each revolution (meters per revolution), and it is a constant for each type of cycle ergometer. The Monark cycle ergometer has a 6 m · rev^{-1} ratio. This means that the flywheel on the Monark cycle will travel 6 m with every complete revolution of the pedals (the flywheel is 1.62 m in circumference and travels 3.7 circuits per pedal revolution). If another brand of cycle is used, then the flywheel travel distance needs to be verified.

Therefore, taking these variables into account, work output can be calculated as:

$$\text{Work output (kg} \cdot \text{m}^{-1} \cdot \text{min}^{-1}) = \text{resistance (kg)} \times \text{cadence (rpm)} \times \text{distance (rpm)}$$

Because the cadence is typically standardized to 50 rpm on the Monark cycle, the participant will always be covering 300 m · min^{-1} (50 rpm × 6 m · rev^{-1}). Examples of some common cycle ergometer work output calculations using the Monark cycle at 50 rpm are as follows:

$$\text{Resistance setting of 1.0 kg: 1.0 kg} \times 50 \text{ rpm} \times 6 \text{ m} \cdot \text{rev}^{-1} = 300 \text{ kg} \cdot \text{m} \cdot \text{min}^{-1}$$

$$\text{Resistance setting of 1.5 kg: 1.5 kg} \times 50 \text{ rpm} \times 6 \text{ m} \cdot \text{rev}^{-1} = 450 \text{ kg} \cdot \text{m} \cdot \text{min}^{-1}$$

$$\text{Resistance setting of 2.0 kg: 2.0 kg} \times 50 \text{ rpm} \times 6 \text{ m} \cdot \text{rev}^{-1} = 600 \text{ kg} \cdot \text{m} \cdot \text{min}^{-1}$$

In addition, it is also important to understand another unit called watts, which is used to express work output. Watts can be determined from kg · m · min^{-1} by dividing by 6.12 (usually rounded to 6). For example, 600 kg · m · min^{-1} is approximately equal to 100 W (600/6.12 = 98 W).

The recommended general procedures for submaximal CRF testing are provided in Box 4.2. It is important to ensure that the participant maintains a constant pedal rate throughout the test (*e.g.*, 50 (±2) rpm). During each work stage, an HRss should be achieved. A HRss is defined as two consecutive HR readings within 6 bpm of each other during one stage. If the HR has increased more than 6 bpm, this indicates the participant has not reached steady state and the stage should be extended for another minute. The resistance setting of the cycle ergometer should be checked regularly throughout the test and corrected if necessary. Even though exercise BP measurements are not required for the computation of CRF, it is suggested that BP is taken and recorded during each stage of the test. These data would be used to end a test early in the event a participant has a hypertensive or hypotensive response.

Åstrand-Ryhming Cycle Ergometer Test

Developed in 1954, the Åstrand-Ryhming cycle ergometer test was developed by Swedish physiologists Per-Olof Åstrand and Irma Ryhming to predict CRF (20). In this submaximal test, the participant is

TABLE 4.2 • Åstrand Cycle Submaximal Cycle Ergometer Test Initial Workloads

Participant	Work Output (kp · m^{-1} · min^{-1})
Men	
Unconditioned	300-600
Conditioned	600-900
Women	
Unconditioned	300-450
Conditioned	450-600
Poorly conditioned or older participants	300

This protocol table is designed as a guide. The protocol is designed to elicit a heart rate (HR) between 125 and 170 bpm by 6 minutes. You can adjust the work output as necessary during the test (usually after the first 6 min) to achieve an HR in or near this range in your subject.

Adapted from American College of Sports Medicine. *ACSM's Health-Related Physical Fitness Assessment Manual.* 2nd ed. Philadelphia, PA: Wolters Kluwer Health Ltd; 2005:121.

asked to complete one 6-minute exercise bout of a standardized work rate — selected according to the recommendations provided in Table 4.2 — to establish a single HRss. At the end of the 6-minute bout, exercise HR is recorded and is expected to be between 125 and 170 bpm, representing 50% and 70% of maximal capacity, respectively. If the HR is below 125 bpm, then workload is increased, and the test continues for an additional 6 minutes.

Estimating $\dot{V}O_{2max}$ using Cycle Ergometer Tests

There are two methods used to derive an estimate of CRF: one involves plotting the data on a graph called a nomogram, and the other uses a calculation-based formula.

Nomogram Technique

A nomogram is a graphic representation where two known data points are plotted and connected with a line to predict a third, unknown value. Figure 4.5 depicts a nomogram used for calculating the unknown $\dot{V}O_{2max}$ from the HR during submaximal work (7). Using this nomogram technique, a mark is placed on the HR scale (left side of nomogram) at the HRss (value between 125 and 170 bpm). Note that this scale actually has two sides, one for men (left) and one for women (right). Next, a mark is placed on the workload scale (right side of nomogram). Note that this scale also has two sides, one for men (right) and one for women (left). The two points are connected with a straight line, and the $\dot{V}O_{2max}$ is read from the center scale. The correction factor table found in Table 4.3 must then be used to adjust the $\dot{V}O_{2max}$ for the person's age (nearest 5 years). For example, if the $\dot{V}O_{2max}$ was estimated to be 3.65 L · min^{-1} from the nomogram, the corrected value for a 40-year-old man would be 3.03 L · min^{-1} (3.65 × 0.83).

TABLE 4.3 • Age Correction Factor for Åstrand Cycle Ergometer Test Results

Age	Correction Factor
15	1.10
25	1.00
35	0.87
40	0.83
45	0.78
50	0.75
55	0.71
60	0.68
65	0.65

Adapted from American College of Sports Medicine. *ACSM's Health-Related Physical Fitness Assessment Manual.* 2nd ed. Philadelphia, PA: Wolters Kluwer Health Ltd; 2005:121.

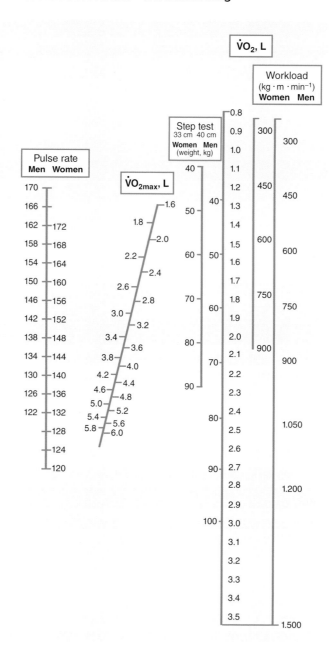

Figure 4.5 Modified Åstrand-Ryhming nomogram. Source: From Åstrand P-O, Ryhming I. A nomogram for calculation of aerobic capacity [physical fitness] from pulse rate during submaximal work. *J Appl Physiol.* 1954;7:218–221, with permission.

Calculation-Based Formula

To calculate the $\dot{V}O_{2max}$ $(mL \cdot kg^{-1} \cdot min^{-1})$ from the single-stage Åstrand-Ryhming protocol, the following formula is used:

$$\dot{V}O_2 = \dot{V}O_21 \times [(220 - age - 73 - (sex \times 10))]/[HR - 73 - (sex \times 10)]$$

where

$\dot{V}O_21$ (submaximal workload) = [(1.8 × work rate)/body weight in kilograms] + 7

Sex = 0 for women and 1 for men

HR = HRss in bpm

For example, $\dot{V}O_{2max}$ for a 33-year-old conditioned woman (63 kg) with a single stage of 600 kg · m⁻¹ · min⁻¹ where the HR value was 134 bpm is given as follows:

Solve for $\dot{V}O_21$:

$$\dot{V}O_21 \ (mL \cdot kg^{-1} \cdot min^{-1}) = [(1.8 \times work\ rate)/body\ weight\ in\ kilograms] + 7$$

$$\dot{V}O_21 \ (mL \cdot kg^{-1} \cdot min^{-1}) = [(1.8 \times 600)/63] + 7 = 24.1$$

Then, inserting $\dot{V}O_2l$ and appropriate sex, age, and HR values into the formula the following value is obtained:

$$\dot{V}O_{2max}\ (mL \cdot kg^{-1} \cdot min^{-1}) = \dot{V}O_2l\ [(220 - age - 73 - (sex \times 10))]/[HR - 73 - (sex \times 10)]$$

$$= 24.1 \times [(220 - 33 - 73 - (0 \times 10))]/[134 - 73 - (0 \times 10)]$$

$$= 45.0\ mL \cdot kg^{-1} \cdot min^{-1}$$

Although the Åstrand-Ryhming is a single-stage test to predict CRF, there are other submaximal tests that include multiple stages, such as the YMCA cycle ergometer test.

The YMCA Cycle Ergometer Test

The protocol for the YMCA cycle ergometer test involves a branching, multistage format that allows to establish a relationship between HR and work rate, to ultimately estimate CRF (10).

The YMCA cycle ergometer test consists of four 3-minute stages at incremental workloads, based on the participants' HR response (Figure 4.6). The completion of the test requires completion of two separate 3-minute stages that result in HR values between 110 and 150 bpm. The test is typically completed between 6 and 12 minutes. Each stage requires the participant to pedal at a constant pedal rate of 50 rpm on a Monark cycle ergometer (10). Stage 1 requires participants to pedal against 0.5 kg of resistance (25 W; 150 kg · m · min^{-1}). The resistance of stage 2 will depend on the participant's steady-state response measured during the last 2 minutes of stage 1.

- HR <80 bpm — change the resistance to 2.5 kg (stage 2; 125 W; 750 kg · m · min^{-1})
- HR 80 to 89 bpm — change the resistance to 2.0 kg (stage 2; 100 W; 600 kg · m · min^{-1})
- HR 90 to 100 bpm — change the resistance to 1.5 kg (stage 2; 75 W; 450 kg · m · min^{-1})
- HR >100 bpm — change the resistance to 1.0 kg (stage 2; 50 W; 300 kg · m · min^{-1})

Use stages 3 and 4 as needed to elicit two consecutive HRss recordings between 110 and 150 bpm. For stages 3 and 4, the resistance used in stage 2 is increased by 0.5 kg (25 W; 150 kg · m · min^{-1}) per stage. Normative tables for the YMCA protocol are published elsewhere (10).

Estimating $\dot{V}O_{2max}$ from the YMCA Cycle Ergometer Test

Similar to the Åstrand-Ryhming cycle ergometer test, there are two methods that can be used to derive an estimate of CRF from a submaximal multistage assessment. One involves plotting the data on a graph and using an extrapolation technique, and the other uses a calculation-based formula.

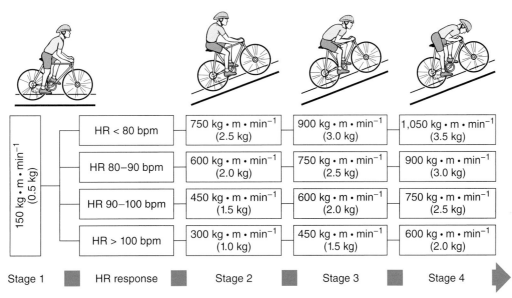

- Speed begins and remains constant throughout test at 50 rpm.
- Each stage is 3-min long.
- Steady-state HR should be achieved (two HRS within 6 bpm) before moving to next stage. If not steady state at the end of stage, add additional 1 min.

Figure 4.6 Cycle ergometer test sequence based on YMCA protocols. HR, heart rate.

Graphing Technique

The graphing method requires that two HR measures be plotted on a graph like the one provided in Figure 4.7. First, a horizontal line is drawn across the graph to intersect the y-axis (HR) at the value of APMHR. Then, a straight line connecting the two highest HR points is drawn. This line is extended (extrapolated) up to the horizontal line that depicts the APMHR. Lastly, a perpendicular line is drawn down from the point of intersection between the APMHR line and the extrapolated line from the achieved HR response to the x-axis (work rate). This work rate value is then the predicted maximal work rate and is used in ACSM metabolic equation for leg cycling to calculate a predicted $\dot{V}O_{2max}$.

$$\dot{V}O_2 \ (mL \cdot kg^{-1} \cdot min^{-1}) = [(1.8 \times \text{work rate})/\text{body weight in kilogram}] + 7$$

Figure 4.8 demonstrates the process of graphing the HR response for prediction of $\dot{V}O_{2max}$. This figure also contains an example of how the inaccuracy of . . . APMHR might influence the results. . . . Thus, it is important that an appropriate equation be used to estimate APMHR.

Calculation-Based Formula

To calculate a predicted $\dot{V}O_{2max}$, it is necessary to first calculate the slope of the HR and $\dot{V}O_2$ relationship. The slope (a) will then be used within a standard linear regression equation of the form $y = ax + b$, where the y variable represents $\dot{V}O_2$ and the x variable represents HR.

Calculation of slope:

$$\text{Slope} \ (a) = (\dot{V}O_22 - \dot{V}O_21)/(HR2 - HR1)$$

where

$\dot{V}O_21$ = submaximal predicted $\dot{V}O_2$ from stage 1, in $mL \cdot kg^{-1} \cdot min^{-1}$
$\dot{V}O_22$ = submaximal predicted $\dot{V}O_2$ from stage 2, in $mL \cdot kg^{-1} \cdot min^{-1}$
$HR1$ = HR from stage 1, in bpm
$HR2$ = HR from stage 2, in bpm

$\dot{V}O_{2max}$ is then estimated from the following equation:

$$\dot{V}O_{2max} \ (mL \cdot kg^{-1} \cdot min^{-1}) = a \ (HR_{max} - HR2) + \dot{V}O_22$$

where

$HR_{max} = 208 - (0.7 \times \text{age})$

For example, a 30-year-old male (75 kg) completed two stages (450 and 600 $kg \cdot m \cdot min^{-1}$) with HR values of 116 and 130 bpm, respectively. His $\dot{V}O_{2max}$ would be calculated as follows:

$$HR_{max} = 208 - (0.7 \times 30) \text{ bpm}$$
$$= 208 - 21$$
$$= 187 \text{ bpm}$$
$$\dot{V}O_21 \ (mL \cdot kg^{-1} \cdot min^{-1}) = [(1.8 \times \text{work rate})/(\text{body weight in kilograms})] + 7$$
$$= [(1.8 \times 450)/75] + 7 = 17.8$$
$$\dot{V}O_22 \ (mL \cdot kg^{-1} \cdot min^{-1}) = [(1.8 \times \text{work rate})/(\text{body weight in kilograms})] + 7$$
$$= [(1.8 \times 600)/75] + 7 = 21.4$$
$$a = (21.4 - 17.8)/(130 - 116) = 0.257$$
$$\dot{V}O_{2max} \ (mL \cdot kg^{-1} \cdot min^{-1}) = a \times (HR_{max} - HR2) + \dot{V}O_22$$
$$= 0.257 \times (187 - 130) + 21.4$$
$$= 36.0 \ mL \cdot kg^{-1} \cdot min^{-1}$$

Recently, a new equation has been proposed to estimate $\dot{V}O_{2max}$, which provides a valid and reliable measure ($R = 0.79$, $R = 0.62$, SEE = 6.6 $mL \cdot kg^{-1} \cdot min^{-1}$) (21). The equation, formulated using over 10,000 individuals between the ages of 20 and 85 years, was created utilizing cycle ergometer and

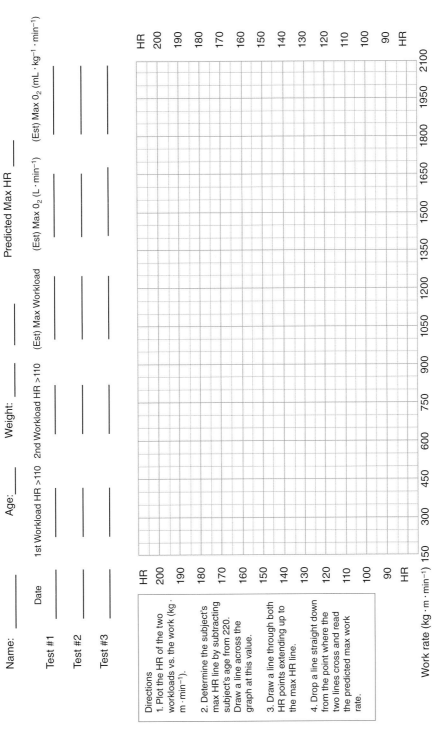

Figure 4.7 A graph used for the prediction of $\dot{V}O_{2max}$ from cycle ergometer tests. HR, heart rate.

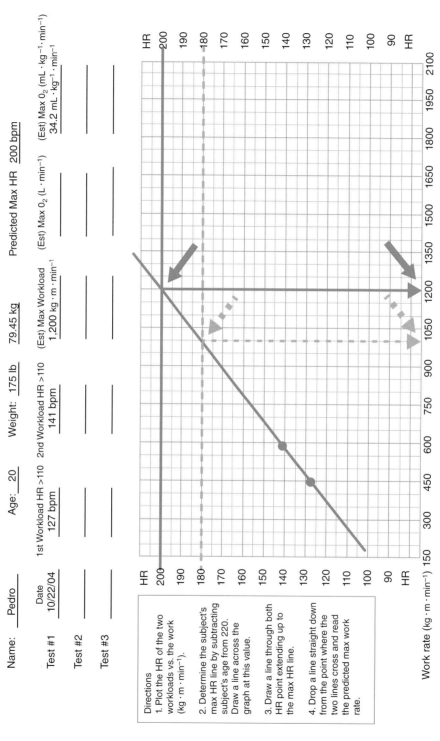

Name: _____Pedro_____

Test #1

Test #2

Test #3

Date
10/22/04

Age: _20_

1st Workload HR >110
127 bpm

Weight: _175 lb_

2nd Workload HR >110
141 bpm

79.45 kg

(Est) Max Workload
1,200 kg · m · min⁻¹

Predicted Max HR _200 bpm_

(Est) Max O₂ (L · min⁻¹)

(Est) Max O₂ (mL · kg⁻¹ · min⁻¹)
34.2 mL · kg⁻¹ · min⁻¹

Directions
1. Plot the HR of the two workloads vs. the work (kg · m · min⁻¹).

2. Determine the subject's max HR line by subtracting subject's age from 220. Draw a line across the graph at this value.

3. Draw a line through both HR point extending up to the max HR line.

4. Drop a line straight down from the point where the two lines cross and read the predicted max work rate.

Figure 4.8 Description of the process of graphing the heart rate (HR) response for the prediction of $\dot{V}O_{2max}$.

treadmill data and can be used with either modality including basic demographic information (21). The proposed equation is:

$$\dot{V}O_{2max} \ (mL \cdot kg^{-1} \cdot min^{-1}) = 45.2 - 0.35 \ (age) - 10.9 \ (sex) - 0.15 \ (weight) + 0.68 \ (height) - 0.46 \ (exercise \ mode)$$

where
  Sex = male = 1; female = 2
  Weight = in pounds
  Height = in inches
  Exercise mode = treadmill = 1; bike = 2

Treadmill

A submaximal treadmill exercise test can also be used to predict CRF. In these tests, the same basic principle of determining the specific linear relationship between HR and $\dot{V}O_2$ is used to derive the predicted values.

Although there are many different treadmill protocols, as will be discussed in Chapter 5, a common one used for submaximal assessments is the Bruce protocol. Most participants should be able to obtain two HR values between 110 and 150 bpm within the first three stages (each 3 min in duration) of this protocol. (Note that the entire Bruce protocol is found in Chapter 5, Table 5.3.)

The basic procedures are identical to the YMCA submaximal cycle protocol with the exception of the mode of exercise. The warm-up minute is performed at 1.7 mph with no elevation. If the participant's HR is ≥110 bpm at stage 1, then only one additional stage is required. Thus, this test typically lasts between 6 and 9 minutes.

Each stage of the Bruce protocol is 3-minutes, and the participant should attempt to complete all 3 minutes of each stage. The participant's HR would be taken every minute throughout each stage. For subsequent measurements, the concept of steady state should apply (two consecutive HR recordings within 6 bpm). If the participant does not achieve steady state by the third minute (which is very possible), then continue to have the participant walk at that same stage for another minute. RPE and BP could also be measured during this protocol, as in the YMCA or Åstrand-Ryhming protocols.

The participant should complete all three stages. The first stage is considered a warm-up stage. The HRss should be between 110 and 150 bpm (some suggest not allowing the HR to exceed 135 bpm) for the last two stages. To predict the maximal aerobic capacity, the following approach would be used:

Estimating $\dot{V}O_{2max}$ from treadmill test

$$\dot{V}O_{2max} \ (mL \cdot kg^{-1} \cdot min^{-1}) = a \times (HR_{max} - HR2) + \dot{V}O_2 2$$

However, the work rate value is now derived from speed (S) and grade (G) on the treadmill and is used in ACSM metabolic equation to calculate a predicted $\dot{V}O_2$:

$$\dot{V}O_2 2 \ (mL \cdot kg^{-1} \cdot min^{-1}) = [(0.1 \times S) + (1.8 \times S \times G)] + 3.5$$

where
  S (speed) = $m \cdot min^{-1}$ (1 mph = 26.8 $m \cdot min^{-1}$)
  G (grade) = % elevation/100

For example, stage 1 with a speed of 1.7 mph and a grade of 10% would have a predicted $\dot{V}O_2$ for this stage calculated as follows:

$$\dot{V}O_2 2 \ (mL \cdot kg^{-1} \cdot min^{-1}) = [(0.1 \times [1.7 \times 26.8]) + (1.8 \times [1.7 \times 26.8] \times [10/100])] + 3.5$$

$$= 16.2 \ mL \times kg^{-1} \cdot min^{-1}$$

INTERPRETATION

Normative values for estimated $\dot{V}O_{2max}$ from the YMCA submaximal cycle ergometer test can be found outside this text and have specific reference to age and sex (10). As indicated earlier, the gold standard test for CRF is a maximal exercise test with $\dot{V}O_{2max}$ measured from the collection of expired gases.

Because both field tests and submaximal exercise tests require prediction of $\dot{V}O_{2max}$, the interpretation of the results needs to include an expression of SEE. Unfortunately, some of the prediction equations used do not provide a SEE. Nonetheless, despite differences in test accuracy and methodology, submaximal testing should be conducted to establish a participant's baseline CRF and used to track relative progress during exercise training.

Moreover, it is important to remember that accurate estimate of $\dot{V}O_{2max}$ is achieved from the HR response to submaximal exercise tests; thus, it is important to make sure the following are achieved before or throughout the test (22):

- A HRss is obtained for each exercise work rate (within ±6 beats).
- A linear relationship exists between HR and work rate.
- The difference between actual and predicted HR_{max} is minimal.
- Mechanical efficiency (*i.e.*, $\dot{V}O_2$ at a given work rate) is the same for everyone.
- Participant is not on any HR altering medications (*e.g.*, β-blockers).
- Participant limits caffeine consumption prior to testing, is not ill, or in a high-temperature environment, all of which may alter the HR response.

Sources of Error in Submaximal Prediction

There are several potential sources of error in submaximal exercise tests when predicting $\dot{V}O_{2max}$ (23,24). Certainly, any errors in the measurement of workload (this would include using an ergometer that was not properly calibrated) or in the measurement of HR will result in prediction error.

One primary source of error is that associated with APMHR. This variability between participants was covered earlier, and an example of the potential for error can be seen in Figure 4.8 by observing the difference in predicted maximal work rate if the actual HR_{max} was 180 bpm (dash lines). As stated, the linear relationship between HR and $\dot{V}O_{2max}$ may be an oversimplification of the actual HR and $\dot{V}O_2$ relationship, as this relationship may be curvilinear near maximum values. This means some participants may have larger increases in $\dot{V}O_2$ compared to the increase in HR as they approach maximum (19), which will impact $\dot{V}O_{2max}$ estimates. A second source of error is the variability in mechanical efficiency on an ergometer. This means, some people will be more efficient at any given workload, requiring less $\dot{V}O_2$ to perform a given work rate. It is estimated that the intersubject variability in measured $\dot{V}O_2$ may have a SEE as high as 7% (25,26). Moreover, some evidence suggests prediction of $\dot{V}O_{2max}$ from submaximal HR is general between 10% and 20% of a person's actual $\dot{V}O_{2max}$. A third source of error is the variability in submaximal HR at the same work rate on different days. One study by Davies (27) reported that at intensities producing HR between 120 and 150 bpm, the HR varied by $\pm8\%$ on different days (19). This is notable because this is the recommended HR range (110–150 bpm) for the YMCA cycle ergometer protocol.

Keeping these limitations in mind, if the primary goal of the test is to determine the change in CRF, it is generally accepted that these serial test results may be useful to document change. Certainly, these changes can be observed from the changes in basic test measurements (test time, HR, and workload) between the tests. If, for example, the HRs at the same stage of a submaximal exercise test were lower, or if the person were able to perform at a higher workload prior to reaching the test termination criteria (*i.e.*, 85% APMHR), this would indicate improved CRF.

SUMMARY

CRF is an important component of physical fitness and one that is commonly desired by participants. Because the measurement of $\dot{V}O_{2max}$ is limited by factors such as time required, cost, and availability of trained personnel, field tests and submaximal exercise tests are frequently performed. As with other fitness measures obtained via prediction equations, appropriate care is needed in interpreting results when CRF is obtained by an estimation method.

LABORATORY ACTIVITIES

Field Test Assessments of Cardiorespiratory Fitness

Data Collection

Form groups of three. Each person is required to do the Queens College step test and one of the following field tests to estimate CRF: 1.5-mi run, 12-minute run/walk, or 1-mi walk. Follow the instructions for each test provided in this chapter.

Laboratory Report

1. Provide the data collected for each test in a summary table along with calculations to estimate CRF from the two field tests.
2. Provide an interpretation of your estimated $\dot{V}O_{2max}$.
3. Discuss possible reasons for the differences in CRF estimates between tests.

Submaximal Exercise Test Assessments of Cardiorespiratory Fitness

Data Collection

Form groups of three. One person in the group will do the YMCA cycle test, one person will do the Åstrand-Ryhming cycle, and one person will do the Bruce treadmill test. Follow the instructions for each test provided in this chapter.

Laboratory Report

1. Provide the data collected for each test in a summary table along with calculations to estimate CRF from the three tests. Note that you need to perform both the graphing method and the calculation method to estimate $\dot{V}O_{2max}$.
2. Provide an interpretation of your estimated $\dot{V}O_{2max}$.
3. Discuss possible reasons for the differences in CRF estimates between this test and the field tests you performed in the previous lab.
4. Which of the preceding tests do you feel best estimates your fitness level and why?

REFERENCES

1. Ross R, Blair SN, Arena R, et al. Importance of assessing cardiorespiratory fitness in clinical practice: a case for fitness as a clinical vital sign: a scientific statement from the American Heart Association. *Circulation*. 2016;134(24):e653–99. doi:10.1161/cir.0000000000000461.
2. Ainsworth BE, Haskell WL, Whitt MC, et al. Compendium of physical activities: an update of activity codes and MET intensities. *Med Sci Sports Exerc*. 2000;32(suppl 9):S498–504. doi:10.1097/00005768-200009001-00009.
3. Tashiro H, Tanaka A, Ishii H, et al. Reduced exercise capacity and clinical outcomes following acute myocardial infarction. *Heart Vessels*. 2020;35(8):1044–50. doi:10.1007/s00380-020-01576-2.
4. Myers J, McAuley P, Lavie CJ, Despres J-P, Arena R, Kokkinos P. Physical activity and cardiorespiratory fitness as major markers of cardiovascular risk: their independent and interwoven importance to health status. *Prog Cardiovasc Dis*. 2015;57(4):306–14. doi:10.1016/j.pcad.2014.09.011.
5. Bennett H, Parfitt G, Davison K, Eston R. Validity of submaximal step tests to estimate maximal oxygen uptake in healthy adults. *Sports Med*. 2016;46(5):737–50. doi:10.1007/s40279-015-0445-1.
6. Jankowski M, Niedzielska A, Brzezinski M, Drabik J. Cardiorespiratory fitness in children: a simple screening test for population studies. *Pediatr Cardiol*. 2015;36(1):27–32. doi:10.1007/s00246-014-0960-0.
7. Åstrand I. Aerobic work capacity in men and women with special reference to age. *Acta Physiol Scand Suppl*. 1960;49(169):1–92.
8. Montoye HJ. The Harvard step test and work capacity. *Rev Can Biol*. 1953;11(5):491–9.
9. McArdle W, Katch F, Pechar G, Jacobson L, Ruck S. Reliability and interrelationships between maximal oxygen intake, physical work capacity and step-test scores in college women. *Med Sci Sports*. 1972;4(4):182–6.
10. YMCA of the USA. In: Golding LA, editor. *YMCA Fitness Testing and Assessment Manual*. Champaign: Human Kinetics; 2000. 247 p.
11. Webb C, Vehrs PR, George JD, Hager R. Estimating VO_{2max} using a personalized step test. *Meas Phys Educ Exerc Sci*. 2014;18(3):184–97. doi:10.1080/1091367X.2014.912985.

12. Knight E, Stuckey MI, Petrella RJ. Validation of the step test and exercise prescription tool for adults. *Can J Diabetes.* 2014;38(3):164–71.

13. Kline GM, Porcari JP, Hintermeister R, et al. Estimation of VO_{2max} from a one-mile track walk, gender, age, and body weight. *Med Sci Sports Exerc.* 1987;19(3):253–9.

14. Maldonado-Martin S, Brubaker PH, Eggebeen J, Stewart KP, Kitzman DW. Association between 6-minute walk test distance and objective variables of functional capacity after exercise training in elderly heart failure patients with preserved ejection fraction: a randomized exercise trial. *Arch Phys Med Rehabil.* 2017;98(3):600–3. doi:10.1016/j.apmr.2016.08.481.

15. Kenney WL, Wilmore JH, Costill DL. Cardiorespiratory responses to acute exercise. In: *Physiology of Sport and Exercise.* Champaign: Human Kinetics; 2020. p. 198–226.

16. Borg GA. *Borg's Perceived Exertion and Pain Scales.* Champaign: Human Kinetics; 1998. 104 p.

17. Fox SM, Naughton JP, Haskell WL. Physical activity and the prevention of coronary heart disease. *Ann Clin Res.* 1971;3(6):404–32.

18. Tanaka H, Monahan KD, Seals DR. Age-predicted maximal heart rate revisited. *J Am Coll Cardiol.* 2001;37(1):153–6. doi:10.1016/s0735-1097(00)01054-8.

19. Achten J, Jeukendrup AE. Heart rate monitoring. *Sports Med.* 2003;33(7):517–38.

20. Åstrand P-O, Ryhming I. A nomogram for calculation of aerobic capacity (physical fitness) from pulse rate during submaximal work. *J Appl Physiol.* 1954;7(2):218–21.

21. de Souza ESCG, Kaminsky LA, Arena R, et al. A reference equation for maximal aerobic power for treadmill and cycle ergometer exercise testing: analysis from the FRIEND registry. *Eur J Prev Cardiol.* 2018;25(7):742–50. doi:10.1177/2047487318763958.

22. Gibson AL, Wagner DR, Heyward VH. Principles of assessment, prescription, and exercise program adherence. In: *Advanced Fitness Assessment and Exercise Prescription.* 8th ed. Champaign: Human Kinetics; 2019. p. 56–76.

23. Åstrand P-O, Rodahl K, Dahl HA, Strømme SB. *Textbook of Work Physiology: Physiological Bases of Exercise.* 4th ed. Champaign: Human Kinetics; 2003.

24. McArdle WD, Katch FI, Katch VL. *Exercise Physiology: Nutrition, Energy, and Human Performance.* Philadelphia (PA): Wolters Kluwer Health/Lippincott Williams & Wilkins; 2015.

25. Katch VL, Sady SS, Freedson P. Biological variability in maximum aerobic power. *Med Sci Sports Exerc.* 1982;14(1):21–5.

26. Noonan V, Dean E. Submaximal exercise testing: clinical application and interpretation. *Phys Ther.* 2000;80(8):782–807.

27. Davies C. Limitations to the prediction of maximum oxygen intake from cardiac frequency measurements. *J Appl Physiol.* 1968;24(5):700–6.

CHAPTER OUTLINE

MAXIMAL EXERCISE TESTING

Estimates of cardiorespiratory fitness (CRF) can be obtained from submaximal exercise tests. However, maximal exercise tests to determine CRF are preferred when greater accuracy is needed to maximize the benefits of an exercise program, or in a clinical setting where treatment decisions are influenced by the test results. CRF in combination with other exercise test measurements can provide valuable clinical information, both prognostic and diagnostic, for participants with and without chronic diseases. This chapter mainly focuses on the procedures used in performing maximal exercise tests in a fitness setting. However, at times, discussion includes topics related to clinical testing for additional context. The reader is encouraged to review the *American College of Sports Medicine (ACSM) Guidelines for Exercise Testing and Prescription, eleventh edition (GETP11)* for more detailed information on performing maximal exercise tests in a clinical setting (1). Several factors are involved in determining when it is appropriate to perform a maximal exercise test in a fitness setting versus a clinical setting. This chapter provides an overview of the personnel training requirements for those performing maximal exercise tests, as well as introduction to testing procedures most commonly utilized.

RISKS

Physical activity and exercise are usually associated with positive health outcomes; however, as previously discussed in Chapter 2, there are potential risks associated with exercise. In general, the risk associated with exercise testing increases with the intensity of the exercise; thus, maximal exercise testing involves a higher degree of risk than other physical fitness assessments (*e.g.*, submaximal exercise tests). Chapter 2 in this text provides an overview of these risks. The reader is referred to the *ACSM's GETP11* for a more in-depth review of the risks associated with exercise and exercise testing. Table 5.1 provides a summary of studies evaluating the risk associated with exercise testing. Moreover, prior to beginning any assessment, it is important to note that the participant has provided consent and that a PAR-Q+ has been completed as a screening tool, at a minimum.

Contraindications

It is essential to ensure that the screening process employed rules out the presence of any absolute or relative contraindications prior to allowing the participant to perform an exercise test. Particular attention should be given to Box 5.1, which provides the contraindications for exercise testing. In a health and fitness setting, any sign or symptom suggestive of underlying disease should be considered a relative contraindication by the health and fitness professional.

TABLE 5.1 • Cardiac Complications During Exercise Testing[a]

References	Year	Site	Number of Tests	MI	VF	Death	Hospitalization	Comment
Rochmis and Blackburn (2)	1971	73 U.S. centers	170,000	NA	NA	1	3	34% of tests were symptom limited; 50% of deaths in 8 h; 50% over the next 4 d
Irving et al. (3)	1977	15 Seattle facilities	10,700	NA	4.67	0	NR	
McHenry (4)	1977	Hospital	12,000	0	0	0	0	
Atterhog et al. (5)	1979	20 Swedish centers	50,000	0.8	0.8	0.4	5.2	
Stuart and Ellestad (6)	1980	1375 U.S. centers	518,448	3.58	4.78	0.5	NR	VF includes other dysrhythmias requiring treatment.
Gibbons et al. (7)	1989	Cooper Clinic	71,914	0.56	0.29	0	NR	Only 4% of men and 2% of women had CVD.
Knight et al. (8)	1995	Geisinger Cardiology Service	28,133	1.42	1.77	0	NR	25% were inpatient tests supervised by non-MDs.
Myers et al. (9)	2000	72 Veterans Affairs Medical Centers in the United States	75,828	0.40	0.13	0	NR	VF includes other dysrhythmias requiring treatment.
Kane et al. (10)	2008	Mayo Clinic	8592	0	4.66	0	5.82	Tests supervised by registered nurses. VF includes other dysrhythmias requiring treatment.

TABLE 5.1 • Cardiac Complications During Exercise Testing[a] (*continued*)

References	Year	Site	Number of Tests	MI	VF	Death	Hospitalization	Comment
Keteyian et al. (11)	2009	82 clinical sites in the United States, Canada, and France	4411	0	0	0	0	All patients diagnosed with heart failure
Skalski et al. (12)	2012	Mayo Clinic	5060	0	7.91	0	11.9	All patients diagnosed with CVD prior to testing. VF includes other dysrhythmias resulting in hospitalization.

[a]Events are per 10,000 tests.

CVD, cardiovascular disease; MD, medical doctor; MI, myocardial infarction; NA, not applicable; NR, not reported; VF, ventricular fibrillation.

From Table 1.4, American College of Sports Medicine. *ACSM's Guidelines for Exercise Testing and Prescription.* 11th ed. Philadelphia, PA: Wolters Kluwer Health Ltd; 2021.

MONITORING

The primary outcome measure of a CRF assessment is the measurement of maximal volume of oxygen ($\dot{V}O_{2max}$) consumed per unit of time ($mL \cdot kg^{-1} \cdot min^{-1}$). This requires measuring the individual's ventilation and the concentrations of oxygen (O_2) and carbon dioxide (CO_2) in the inspired and expired air during the maximal exercise test. Although heart rate (HR) is not required to calculate $\dot{V}O_{2max}$, it is typically measured throughout the maximal exercise test. It is also essential to monitor the participant for signs and symptoms of exercise intolerance, which would indicate early termination of the test. General indications for terminating the test are provided. Chapter 3 of the *ACSM's GETP11* provides detailed instructions related to the assessment of CRF.

Maximal exercise tests are also performed in preventive and rehabilitative exercise program settings. Because the opportunity exists to observe a variety of physiologic responses to exercise, additional monitoring, including exercise electrocardiography (ECG), blood pressure (BP), and measurement of

Box 5.1   Contraindications to Symptom-Limited Maximal Exercise Testing

Absolute Contraindications
- Acute myocardial infarction within 2 days
- Ongoing unstable angina
- Uncontrolled cardiac arrhythmia with hemodynamic compromise
- Active endocarditis
- Symptomatic severe aortic stenosis
- Decompensated heart failure
- Acute pulmonary embolism, pulmonary infarction, or deep venous thrombosis
- Acute myocarditis or pericarditis
- Acute aortic dissection
- Physical disability that precludes safe and adequate testing

Relative Contraindications
- Known obstructive left main coronary artery stenosis
- Moderate-to-severe aortic stenosis with uncertain relationship to symptoms
- Tachyarrhythmias with uncontrolled ventricular rates
- Acquired advanced or complete heart block
- Recent stroke or transient ischemia attack
- Mental impairment with limited ability to cooperate
- Resting hypertension with systolic >200 mm Hg or diastolic >110 mm Hg
- Uncorrected medical conditions, such as significant anemia, important electrolyte imbalance, and hyperthyroidism

Reprinted with permission from Fletcher GF, Ades PA, Kligfield P, et al. Exercise standards for testing and training: a scientific statement from the American Heart Association. *Circulation.* 2013;128(8):873–934. doi:10.1161/CIR.0b013e31829b5b44.

TABLE 5.2 • Recommended Monitoring Intervals for Graded Exercise Testing Outcome Variables

Variable	Before Exercise Test	During Exercise Test	After Exercise Test
ECG	Monitored continuously; recorded supine position and posture of exercise	Monitored continuously; recorded during the last 15 s of each stage (interval protocol) or the last 15 s of each 2-min period (ramp protocols)	Monitored continuously; recorded immediately postexercise, during the last 15 s of first minute of recovery, and then every 2 min thereafter
HR[a,b]	Monitored continuously; recorded supine position and posture of exercise	Monitored continuously; recorded during the last 5 s of each minute	Monitored continuously; recorded during the last 5 s of each minute
BP[a,c]	Measured and recorded in supine position and posture of exercise	Measured and recorded during the last 45 s of each stage (interval protocol) or the last 45 s of each 2-min period (ramp protocols)	Measured and recorded immediately postexercise and then every 2 min thereafter
Signs and symptoms	Monitored continuously; recorded as observed	Monitored continuously; recorded as observed	Monitored continuously; recorded as observed
RPE	Explain scale	Recorded during the last 5 s of each minute	Obtain peak exercise value; then not measured in recovery
Gas exchange	Baseline reading to assure proper operational status	Measured continuously	Generally not needed in recovery

[a] An unchanged or decreasing systolic BP with increasing workloads should be retaken (*i.e.*, verified immediately).

[b] HR is measured via HR monitor if ECG is not available.

[c] In addition, BP and HR should be assessed and recorded whenever adverse symptoms or abnormal ECG changes occur.

BP, blood pressure; ECG, electrocardiogram; HR, heart rate; RPE, ratings of perceived exertion.

Data from Cole CR, Blackstone EH, Pashkow FJ, Snader CE, Lauer MS. Heart rate recovery immediately after exercise as a predictor of mortality. *N Engl J Med*. 1999;341:1351–7.

oxygen saturation, is routinely performed with the assessment of CRF. Chapter 4 of the *ACSM's GETP11* provides a thorough overview of the procedures used in clinical exercise testing settings. Table 5.2 provides recommendations for the monitoring intervals of various measures typically recorded during maximal exercise testing. This monitoring typically requires trained staff and additional equipment, which are common to most clinical exercise facilities.

PERSONNEL

Multiple staff are needed to administer maximal exercise testing, with the exact number being determined by the amount of monitoring used and/or facility standards. The most commonly monitored variables during a maximal exercise test are ECG, HR, metabolic measurements ($\dot{V}O_2$), BP, rating of perceived exertions (RPEs), and, possibly, oxygen saturation. In addition, the work rates of the treadmill or cycle ergometer should be controlled or monitored by the staff if controlled by a computer program.

The purpose of the test and the status of the participant being tested will impact the personnel needed for the test. If the purpose of the test is diagnostic in nature, a physician or other qualified health care provider (nurse practitioner or physician assistant) should be present or easily available. This is the case even if the direct supervision (and even preliminary interpretation) is provided by other appropriately trained health care personnel, including clinical exercise physiologist (CEP). In addition, it is recommended that the nonphysician allied health care professional administering clinical exercise tests should have cognitive skills (see Box 5.2) similar to, although not as extensive as, the physician who provides the final interpretation. Thus, it is accepted that a trained and experienced health care professional, such as an ACSM-CEP with the requisite knowledge, skills, and abilities, can administer

Box 5.2	Cognitive Skills Required to Competently Supervise Exercise Tests

- Knowledge of appropriate indications for exercise testing
- Knowledge of alternative physiologic cardiovascular tests
- Knowledge of appropriate contraindications, risks, and risk assessment of testing
- Knowledge to promptly recognize and treat complications of exercise testing
- Competence in cardiopulmonary resuscitation and successful completion of an American Heart Association–sponsored course in advance cardiovascular life support and renewal on a regular basis
- Knowledge of various exercise protocols and indications for each
- Knowledge of basic cardiovascular and exercise physiology, including hemodynamic response to exercise
- Knowledge of cardiac arrhythmia and the ability to recognize and treat serious arrhythmias
- Knowledge of cardiovascular drugs and how they can affect exercise performance, hemodynamics, and the ECG
- Knowledge of the effects of age and disease on hemodynamic and the electrocardiographic response to exercise
- Knowledge of principles and details of exercise testing, including proper lead placement and skin preparation
- Knowledge of end points of exercise testing and indications to terminate exercise testing

Adapted from Rodgers GP, Ayanian JZ, Balady G, et al. American College of Cardiology/American Heart Association clinical competence statement on stress testing. a report of the American College of Cardiology/American Heart Association/American College of Physicians-American Society of Internal Medicine Task Force on Clinical Competence. *Circulation*. 2000;102(14): 1726–1738. doi:10.1161/01.cir.102.14.1726 (13).

maximal exercise tests (14). Modifications to the exercise test will impact the need for available staff, as healthier participants will require less monitoring, and more experienced staff will be able to complete a greater number of tasks during the test.

In situations where exercise testing is performed, site personnel should at least be certified at a level of basic life support (cardiopulmonary resuscitation) and have automated external defibrillator (AED) training. Preferably, one or more staff members should also be certified in first aid and advanced cardiac life support (15). Moreover, research laboratories and testing facilities should, at a minimum, have access to an AED (as shown in Figure 5.1) and first aid equipment. The facility also needs to have a written set of emergency procedures with a regular schedule of review/practice sessions in which all personnel must participate, as illustrated in Figure 5.2.

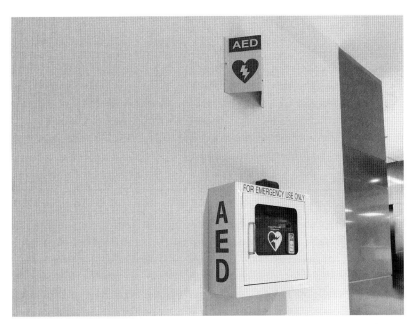

Figure 5.1 An automated external defibrillator (AED) is essential in all physical fitness assessment settings.

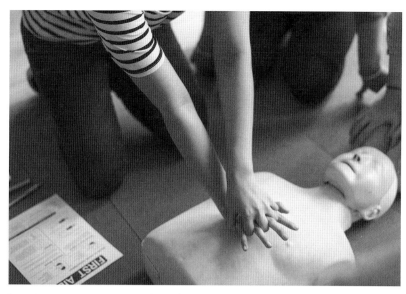

Figure 5.2 Regular emergency procedure drills should include a practice session of cardiopulmonary resuscitation.

Test Operator

Depending on the facility, participants will complete all prescreening documents prior to or immediately before testing (see Chapter 2). In either case, it is important for someone involved during the exercise test to go over these documents and perform a pretest review of the participant's health history, making sure that there are no contraindications for testing. The informed consent document should be reviewed again, providing an opportunity to ask additional questions, and the exercise test procedures should be explained. The test supervisor should ensure the participant understands the nature of the test and that although the objective is to work to a maximal effort level, the test can be stopped at any time, and the staff should be promptly informed if anything unusual is experienced during the test (particularly symptoms of ischemia such as chest discomfort). An explanation of the RPE scale should be provided at this time. The test supervisor may also perform one of the test technician roles during the test.

Staff Responsibilities During Testing

All testing should start with a brief 1- to 2-minute warm-up (treadmill — slow speed of walking; cycle — unloaded pedaling). During this time, the staff should make sure all equipment is functioning properly and that the participant is relatively comfortable on the exercise ergometer. When the staff and the participant are ready, the protocol begins, and the sequence of measures, as described in Table 5.2, is performed. To ensure participant safety, it is important that all staff observe the participant during the test and that one specific staff member is assigned this responsibility as a primary role. In many laboratories, the technician performing the BP measurements will also obtain measures of RPE and become the primary observer and communicator with the participant. One staff member is typically in charge of recording data (HR, BP, RPE, and symptoms) during the test. The technician monitoring the ECG, or other monitor of HR, commonly performs this duty. In addition, one technician monitors the readings from the metabolic measurements and can control the workload changes during the test. This technician would also be responsible for the pretest calibration of the metabolic cart and the posttest cleaning and sterilization of the mouthpiece and breathing valve used by the participant. The staff should provide feedback to the participant throughout the test and encourage a maximal effort. Common objective indicators of maximal effort have been recommended and include (a) a respiratory exchange ratio (RER) of ≥ 1.1; (b) a plateau in volume of oxygen consumed per unit time ($\dot{V}O_2$)

— no further increase in $\dot{V}O_2$ with an increase in work rate; and (c) achievement of age-predicted maximal HR (HR_{max}). It is worth noting that these objective indicators have been challenged (16), suggesting they may not be suitable to determine $\dot{V}O_{2max}$, as reliance in them may underestimate this measure between 30% and 40%. Subjective indicators of maximal effort typically include an RPE measurement (17). Using the original Borg scale, (6–20) a rating >18 indicates the participant has reached maximal effort (18), and values above 15 suggest the participant is working above their ventilatory threshold (18).

SELECTING THE MODE FOR TESTING

The most common modes for exercise testing are the treadmill and the cycle ergometer. These two modes are commonly used because of the ability to easily replicate and control work rates. Arm ergometers, which also have the ability to replicate and control work rates, are used for participants with disabilities that prevent or limit the use of their legs.

For several reasons, the default, or standard, selection for maximal exercise testing is the treadmill. In the United States, there is more experience with treadmill testing; and for most people, walking is the most common form of daily movement, thus making walking on a treadmill somewhat more comfortable than a cycle ergometer. Generally, treadmill exercise tests produce higher $\dot{V}O_{2max}$ values than tests on cycle ergometers because the relative unfamiliarity with cycling often results in local muscular fatigue. Unless compelling reasons exist to suggest otherwise, the choice for exercise mode is typically the treadmill.

The cycle ergometer may be the preferred mode in certain situations. If the participant were a trained cyclist or desire to exercise primarily on a cycle ergometer, then a cycle test would be appropriate. The cycle might also be selected if the participant has a disability, injury, or health condition that would make walking difficult or that could actually be worsened by walking. Participants who are obese may be better served by a cycle ergometer because it is designed to support body weight, as opposed to the treadmill in which the participant's body must support all weight. Other reasons for selecting a cycle ergometer may be related to facility constraints, such as space and power supply. The cycle ergometer also costs less, is more portable, and operates more quietly than a treadmill.

PROTOCOLS

Once the decision on mode of exercise is made, the testing supervisor needs to determine which test protocol to employ. It is wise to set one standard or default protocol that will be used most typically within a given facility. A standard protocol allows for the monitoring of typical, expected responses during the test as well as for comparisons between tests. Several considerations should be taken into account when altering standard protocols and several principles should guide this process: (a) whether the protocol will result in a maximal effort between 6 and 15 minutes (ideally between 8 and 12 minutes); (b) how to increment the work rate, either in stages or as a slow, continuous increase (ramp style). Another consideration to keep in mind when using treadmill tests is whether the work rate should be increased only through an increase in grade (*i.e.*, a fixed speed protocol) or by increasing both speed and grade. Typically, for more deconditioned participants, increments in grade may be better tolerated than simultaneous changes in speed and grade.

There are many standardized protocols from which to choose, as indicated in Figure 5.3. Ramp protocols increase the workload more gradually, usually by shortening the stage time and decreasing the work rate increments. Although ramp protocols for cycle ergometers have been available for a longer period of time, systems to provide ramping increments for treadmills have only been available since the 1990s. Some facilities choose to individualize the protocol for each participant to reach a target test time associated with a pretest prediction of the participant's $\dot{V}O_{2max}$ based on participant characteristics. Typically, these individualized protocols are determined by a computer program found on some commercial exercise testing systems. It is beyond the scope of this manual to provide a thorough explanation of different protocols, including arm ergometer protocols; however, several commonly used protocols are reviewed.

METs	Cycle Ergometer	Ramp (Per 30 s) mph	%Gr	Modified Bruce 3-min Stages mph	%GR	Bruce 3-min Stages mph	%GR	Naughton 2-min Stages mph	%Gr	Modified Naughton (CHF) 2-min Stages mph	%GR
21	For 70 kg body weight										
20				6.0	22	6.0	22				
19	1 Watt = 6.1 kpm · min⁻¹										
18				5.5	20	5.5	20				
17											
16											
15	kpm · min⁻¹			5.0	18	5.0	18				
14	1500									3.0	25
13	1350	3.0 / 3.0	25.0 / 24.0	4.2	16	4.2	16			3.0	22.5
12		3.0 / 3.0	23.0 / 22.0							3.0	20
11	1200	3.0 / 3.0	21.0 / 20.0							3.0	17.5
10	1050	3.0 / 3.0 / 3.0	19.0 / 18.0 / 17.0	3.4	14	3.4	14			3.0	15
9	900	3.0 / 3.0	16.0 / 15.0					mph / %Gr		3.0	12.5
8		3.0 / 3.0	14.0 / 13.0					2	17.5	3.0	10
7	750	3.0 / 3.0 / 3.0	12.0 / 11.0 / 10.0	2.5	12	2.5	12	2	14.0	3.0	7.5
6	600	3.0 / 3.0 / 3.0	9.0 / 8.0 / 7.0							2.0	10.5
5	450	3.0 / 3.0	6.0 / 5.0	1.7	10	1.7	10	2	10.5	2.0	7.0
4	300	3.0 / 3.0 / 3.0	4.0 / 3.0 / 2.0					2	7.0	2.0	3.5
3	150	3.0 / 2.5	1.0 / 0	1.7	5			2	3.5	1.5	0
2		2.0 / 1.5	0 / 0	1.7	0			2	0	1.0	0
1		1.0 / 0.5	0 / 0					1	0		

Figure 5.3 Common exercise protocols and associated metabolic costs of each stage. CHF, congestive heart failure; METs, metabolic equivalents; %Gr, percent grade. Source: Fletcher GF, Ades PA, Kligfield P, et al. (2013). Exercise standards for testing and training: A scientific statement from the American Heart Association. *Circulation.* 128(8):873–934. doi:10.1161/CIR.0b013e31829b5b44.

Bruce Protocol

Dr. Robert Bruce, a cardiologist, developed the Bruce protocol in 1973 (19). The Bruce protocol is one of the most commonly used protocols in both clinical and nonclinical exercise testing laboratories. Surveys of exercise testing laboratories in the United States have consistently reported the Bruce protocol, or modified versions, to be the one most (82%) commonly used (20). This popularity is in part a result of the substantial amount of data on the typical responses expected with the Bruce protocol, including predictions of $\dot{V}O_{2max}$, based on treadmill time, as reviewed later in this chapter.

The Bruce protocol consists of 3-minute stages where the speed and grade both increase with each stage, and the work rate increment is ~3 metabolic equivalents (METs) per stage. The initial stage of this protocol is set at a MET level of 4.6, which may be too large of a requirement for deconditioned adults, many elderly participants, and patients with cardiac and pulmonary disease. As a result, a modified version of the protocol includes either one or two preliminary stages (stages 0 and 0.5), as indicated in Table 5.3.

Balke-Ware Protocol

Another commonly used treadmill protocol is the Balke-Ware, developed by Dr. Bruno Balke and colleagues (21). The main features of this protocol are that it is of fixed speed (3.3 mph) and the rate of increment in work rate is relatively small (≈0.5 MET) at each stage (1 minute). There have been several modifications made to this protocol, one of which has been employed routinely over the years

TABLE 5.3 • Bruce Treadmill Protocol

Stage	Speed (mph/km · h⁻¹)	Grade (%)
0ᵃ	1.7/2.7	0.0
0.5ᵃ	1.7/2.7	5.0
1	1.7/2.7	10.0
2	2.5/4.0	12.0
3	3.4/5.5	14.0
4	4.2/6.7	16.0
5	5.0/8.0	18.0
6	5.5/8.9	20.0
7	6.0/9.7	22.0

ᵃModified Bruce stages. All stages are 3 minutes in duration. For estimated metabolic equivalent levels, see Figure 5.3 (19).

TABLE 5.4 • Modified Balke-Ware Treadmill Protocol

	Modifiedᵃ		
Stage	Time (min:s)	Speed (mph/km · h⁻¹)	Grade (%)
1	0:00	3.0/4.8	0.0
2	2:00	3.0/4.8	2.5
3	4:00	3.0/4.8	5.0
4	6:00	3.0/4.8	7.5
5	8:00	3.0/4.8	10.0
6	10:00	3.0/4.8	12.5
7	12:00	3.0/4.8	15.0
8	14:00	3.0/4.8	17.5
9	16:00	3.0/4.8	20.0
10	18:00	3.0/4.8	22.5
11	20:00	3.0/4.8	25.0

Original test includes a fixed speed (3.3 mph/5.3 km · h⁻¹) and 1% elevation (starting at 0%) increase every minute until exhaustion.

ᵃThe speed for the modified protocol can be selected to meet the comfort level of the patient. Other common variations are 2.0 and 2.5 mph. For estimated metabolic equivalent levels, see Figure 5.3.

From Balke B, Ware R. An experimental study of physical fitness of Air Force personnel. *US Armed Forces Med J.* 1959;10:675–688.

at the Cooper Clinic in Dallas, Texas. A common modification to the Balke-Ware protocol is given in Table 5.4.

Running Protocols

As the principle of specificity would suggest, trained endurance runners will perform best on a protocol that allows them to run at faster speeds and lower elevations than the treadmill tests described earlier. Obviously, because of the increased noise and body motion associated with running protocols, the ability to obtain and monitor variables such as BP and heart function, with the use of an ECG, will be limited. Thus, these types of protocols are only indicated for healthy participants who run regularly as part of training. Running protocols typically feature a beginning phase where the participant runs at a

TABLE 5.5 • Modified Costill/Fox Running Protocol

Stage	Time (min)	Speed (mph/km · h⁻¹)	Grade (%)
Warm-up	0–4	3.1/5.0	0.0
Speed increasing stages[a]	4 each	5.9/9.5	0.0
		7.5/12.0	
		8.4/13.5	
		9.9/16.0	
Grade increasing stages	2 each		2.0
			4.0
			5.0
			8.0

[a]Speed (4 min per stage) continues to increase until the subject reaches a rating of perceived exertion (RPE) of 13. Then, speed remains constant, and the grade increases by 2% every 2 minutes until exhaustion.
Speeds in mph are 3.1 (warm-up) and 5.9, 7.5, 8.4, and 9.9 (each running speed, respectively).

moderate pace for a couple of minutes to warm up, followed by a rapid increase to the peak sustained running speed desired by the participant. Further increments in work are obtained by making modest increases in grade until the participant reaches maximum capacity. A modified Costill/Fox protocol is presented in Table 5.5 (22).

Cycle Protocols

A cycling protocol involves a non–weight-bearing mode of exercise, and thus, the workload is set by pedaling against an external resistance. The ability to push this resistance will be determined, to a large degree, by the amount of muscle mass a person possesses. Although the absolute level of work is greater for the larger person, CRF is measured in units relative to body weight (*i.e.*, $mL \cdot kg^{-1} \cdot min^{-1}$). Table 5.6 provides one commonly used protocol for cycle testing that uses 2-minute stages with work rate increments of $150 \ kg \cdot m \cdot min^{-1}$. When testing a larger person, the protocol may start with a higher workload or it may use larger increments during the test.

Individualized Protocols

Using an individualized protocol, the general idea is to arrive at a comfortable walking or jogging speed on the treadmill for the participant. This then will be the speed used throughout the entire duration of the test. One way to do this is:

TABLE 5.6 • An Example of a Cycle Test Protocol

Stage	Time (min:s)	Work Rate (kg · m · min⁻¹)
1	0:00	150
2	2:00	300
3	4:00	450
4	6:00	600
5	8:00	750
6	10:00	900
7	12:00	1050
8	14:00	1200

For larger individuals, the work rates may need to be doubled.

1. As an orientation to the treadmill, start the treadmill at a walking speed of around 2.0 mph.
2. When the participant appears to be comfortable, increase the walking speed to approach their normal workout speed. Allow time for your client to adjust to each new treadmill speed. Closely observe the participant to ensure that the speed is appropriate. People will often say they walk/jog faster than they really do. If your client reports to exercise outside by walking or running, then convert the exercise routine into a speed (*i.e.*, they walk about 2.5 miles in 50 minutes; that equals 3 mph), then set the speed of the treadmill slower than this speed. Once again, the key is your client's comfort and appearance.
3. Once a comfortable walking or running speed has been established, use this speed for your test, adjusting the treadmill grade at specific time points (*i.e.*, every 1 minute).
4. An alternative protocol calls for an increase in grade (1% per min) after walking or running speed has been established.

MEASURED AND ESTIMATED $\dot{V}O_{2max}$

To provide the gold-standard measure of CRF, the maximal exercise test must include the assessment of $\dot{V}O_2$ with a metabolic measurement system. These systems will provide measures of exercise ventilation and expired concentrations of O_2 and CO_2 to derive the measurement of $\dot{V}O_{2max}$. These metabolic measurement systems can also provide a detailed recording of the responses throughout the test and can be used to provide other data of interest to the participant (*e.g.*, ventilatory threshold).

The measurement of $\dot{V}O_{2max}$ is not always feasible because metabolic measurement systems are relatively expensive to purchase and to maintain. These systems also require additional expertise of the personnel operating them and interpreting results. When direct measurement is not available, it is possible to predict $\dot{V}O_{2max}$ from either the total time or the peak workload obtained during a maximal exercise test. As with all predicted results, interpretation must include an expression of the error range.

Estimating $\dot{V}O_{2max}$ from Exercise Test Time

Several research reports have provided regression equations to obtain an estimate of $\dot{V}O_{2max}$ from exercise test duration. When using prediction models, it is essential that the identical protocol is followed for the test and that the subject is not allowed to use handrail support during the treadmill test. It is also desirable to match the characteristics of the subject to the general characteristics of the population that was assessed in the original study. Box 5.3 provides prediction equations for the Bruce, BSU/Bruce ramp, and Balke-Ware protocols. Note that the standard error of estimates (SEEs) range from ± 2.7 to $\pm 4.7 \text{ mL} \cdot \text{kg}^{-1} \cdot \text{min}^{-1}$. The reference tables for CRF interpretation (Table 5.7) also provide an estimate for the modified Balke-Ware protocol used at the Cooper Clinic.

Estimating $\dot{V}O_{2max}$ from Peak Workload

Another approach to obtaining an estimate of $\dot{V}O_{2max}$ is to use the ACSM metabolic calculations, which can be found in Chapter 6. However, this method is not desirable because the metabolic calculation equations were developed for steady-state submaximal work rates. However, for cycle testing or other treadmill protocols without prediction equations based on test time, they are sometimes used.

INTERPRETATION

As with other measures, no national standard has been developed and accepted for interpreting CRF. However, ACSM has long used the data developed by the Cooper Clinic in Dallas, Texas, as a source for providing interpretations of CRF assessments. These CRF gender-specific charts are provided in Table 5.7. Similar to the body composition norms, it is important to recognize that these values are based on the population that has received these measures and are expressed as percentiles, which may limit their usefulness for interpreting test results from populations with different characteristics.

Box 5.3	**Examples of Regression Equations for Age-Predicted Normal Standards for Exercise Capacity**

Directly measured versus estimated values are indicated for each equation
Hansen, Sue, and Wasserman equations for measured VO_{2peak} (23):

	Mode	Overweight	Predicted VO_2 max (mL · min^{-1})
Males	Cycle[a]	No	$Wt \times [50.72 - (0.372 \times A)]$
		Yes	$[0.79 \times (Ht - 60.7)] \times [50.72 - (0.372 \times A)]$
	Treadmill[b]	No	$Wt \times [56.36 - (0.413 \times A)]$
		Yes	$[0.79 \times (Ht - 60.7)] \times [56.36 - (0.413 \times A)]$
Females	Cycle[a]	No	$(42.8 + Wt) \times [22.78 - (0.17 \times A)]$
		Yes	$Ht \times [14.81 - (0.11 \times A)]$
	Treadmill[c]	No	$Wt \times [44.37 - (0.413 \times A)]$
		Yes	$[0.79 \times (Ht - 68.2)] \times [44.37 - (0.413 \times A)]$

Wt = weight in kg; Ht = height in cm; A = age in years

[a]Overweight is $Wt > [0.79 \times (Ht - 60.7)]$.

[b]Overweight is $Wt > [0.65 \times (Ht - 42.8)]$.

[c]Overweight is $Wt > [0.79 \times (Ht - 68.2)]$.

Fitness Registry and the Importance of Exercise: A National Data Base (FRIEND) equation for measured VO_{2peak} (24):

$$VO_{2peak} \text{ (mL} \cdot \text{kg}^{-1} \cdot \text{min}^{-1}) = 45.2 - 0.35 \times \text{age} - 10.9 \times \text{gender (male = 1; female = 2)} - 0.15 \times \text{weight (lb)} + 0.68 \times \text{height (in)} - 0.46 \times \text{exercise mode (treadmill = 1; bike = 2)}$$

Percentage exercise capacity achieved in estimated METs among male Veterans (25):

$$\text{All individuals: METs} = 14.7 - 0.11 \text{ (age)}$$

$$\text{Active individuals: METs} = 16.4 - 0.13 \text{ (age)}$$

$$\text{Sedentary individuals: METs} = 11.9 - 0.07 \text{ (age)}$$

Percentage predicted VO_{2peak} in men and women with a medical or surgical diagnosis (mL · kg^{-1} · min^{-1}) (26):

$$\text{Men: } 33.97 - 0.242 \times \text{age}$$

$$\text{Women: } 21.69 - 0.116 \times \text{age}$$

Percentage predicted exercise capacity achieved in healthy women (estimated METs) (27):

$$\text{METs} = 14.7 - (0.13 \times \text{age}).$$

Bruce, Kusumi, and Hosmer (19):

$$\dot{V}O_{2max} = 6.70 - 2.82 \text{ (men = 1, women = 2)} + 0.056 \text{ (time in seconds)}$$

Kaminsky and Whaley (28):

$$\dot{V}O_{2max} = 3.9 \text{ (time in minutes)} - 7.0$$

Pollock et al. (29):

Using the Balke protocol with a standard speed of 3.0 mph/4.8 km · h^{-1}

$$\dot{V}O_{2max} = 0.023 \text{ (time in seconds)} + 5.2$$

Pollock et al. (30)
Using the Balke protocol with a standard speed of 3.3 mph/5.3 km · h^{-1}
$$\dot{V}O_{2max} = 1.444 \text{ (time in minutes)} + 14.99$$

TABLE 5.7 • Treadmill-Based Cardiorespiratory Fitness Classifications ($\dot{V}O_{2max}$) by Age and Sex

		$\dot{V}O_{2max}$ (mL $O_2 \cdot kg^{-1} \cdot min^{-1}$)				
Men		**Age Group (yr)**				
Percentile		20-29	30-39	40-49	50-59	60-69
95	Superior	66.3	59.8	55.6	50.7	43.0
90	Excellent	61.8	56.5	52.1	45.6	40.3
85		59.3	54.2	49.3	43.2	38.2
80		57.1	51.6	46.7	41.2	36.1
75	Good	55.2	49.2	45.0	39.7	34.5
70		53.7	48.0	43.9	38.2	32.9
65		52.1	46.6	42.1	36.3	31.6
60		50.2	45.2	40.3	35.1	30.5
55	Fair	49.0	43.8	38.9	33.8	29.1
50		48.0	42.4	37.8	32.6	28.2
45		46.5	41.3	36.7	31.6	27.2
40		44.9	39.6	35.7	30.7	26.6
35	Poor	43.5	38.5	34.6	29.5	25.7
30		41.9	37.4	33.3	28.4	24.6
25		40.1	35.9	31.9	27.1	23.7
20		38.1	34.1	30.5	26.1	22.4
15	Very poor	35.4	32.7	29.0	24.4	21.2
10		32.1	30.2	26.8	22.8	19.8
5		29.0	27.2	24.2	20.9	17.4
Women						
Percentile		20-29	30-39	40-49	50-59	60-69
95	Superior	56.0	45.8	41.7	35.9	29.4
90	Excellent	51.3	41.4	38.4	32.0	27.0
85		48.3	39.3	36.0	30.2	25.6
80		46.5	37.5	34.0	28.6	24.6
75	Good	44.7	36.1	32.4	27.6	23.8
70		43.2	34.6	31.1	26.8	23.1
65		41.6	33.5	30.0	26.0	22.0
60		40.6	32.2	28.7	25.2	21.2
55	Fair	38.9	31.2	27.7	24.4	20.5
50		37.6	30.2	26.7	23.4	20.0
45		35.9	29.3	25.9	22.7	19.6
40		34.6	28.2	24.9	21.8	18.9
35	Poor	33.6	27.4	24.1	21.2	18.4
30		32.0	26.4	23.3	20.6	17.9
25		30.5	25.3	22.1	19.9	17.2
20		28.6	24.1	21.3	19.1	16.5
15	Very poor	26.2	22.5	20.0	18.3	15.6
10		23.9	20.9	18.8	17.3	14.6
5		21.7	19.0	17.0	16.0	13.4
		(n = 410)	(n = 608)	(n = 843)	(n = 805)	(n = 408)

Percentiles from cardiopulmonary exercise testing on a treadmill with measured $\dot{V}O_{2max}$ (mL $O_2 \cdot kg^{-1} \cdot min^{-1}$). Data obtained from the Fitness Registry and the Importance of Exercise National Database (FRIEND) Registry for men and women who were considered free from known cardiovascular disease.

Adapted with permission from: Kaminsky LA. Imboden MT, Arena R, Myers J. Reference standards for cardiorespiratory fitness measured with cardiopulmonary exercise testing using cycle ergometry: data from the Fitness Registry and the Importance of Exercise National Database (FRIEND) Registry. *Mayo Clin Proc.* 2017;92(2):228-233.

SUMMARY

The gold-standard measure of CRF is the maximal exercise test with measurement of ventilation and the concentrations of O_2 and CO_2 in the inspired and expired air. Because of the increased risks for the participant to perform this high-intensity test, the relatively expensive equipment required to obtain the necessary measurements, and the high level of training required of the testing personnel, this procedure is not routinely performed in all assessment settings. However, fitness professionals working in preventive and rehabilitative exercise programs will often be involved in performing this form of CRF assessment.

LABORATORY ACTIVITIES

Maximal Exercise Tests

Data Collection

The class will perform three maximal exercise tests, one each on three different subjects. One student will perform a BSU/Bruce treadmill protocol, one student will perform a modified Costill/Fox running protocol, and one student will perform a maximal test on a cycle ergometer. Follow the instructions for monitoring and test administration presented in this chapter. For each test, a different group of students will perform the roles of the different technicians.

Laboratory Report

1. Using the exercise test data recording sheet, make a graph for each test of the HR (x-axis) and O_2 (y-axis) relationship.
2. Did all subjects reach a true $\dot{V}O_{2max}$? What objective criteria indicate they did or did not give a maximal effort? Interpret the test results for each subject.
3. For the cycle test, pretend the test was stopped after the subject completed two stages with HR values between 110 and 150 beats per minute (bpm). Use those submaximal data to predict $\dot{V}O_{2max}$ using the methods discussed in Chapter 7. How does this predicted value compare to the measured value from the maximal exercise test?
4. Use the prediction formula based on treadmill test time for the BSU/Bruce ramp test to predict $\dot{V}O_{2max}$. How does this predicted value compare to the measured value from the maximal exercise test?
5. Which submaximal assessment (performed by these subjects in the labs from Chapter 7) predicted actual $\dot{V}O_{2max}$ the best for each subject? Discuss why this particular submaximal test may have been a better predictor than the other tests for that subject.

REFERENCES

1. American College of Sports Medicine. *ACSM's Guidelines for Exercise Testing and Prescription.* 10th ed. Philadelphia (PA): Lippincott Williams & Wilkins; 2017.
2. Rochmis P, Blackburn H. Exercise tests. A survey of procedures, safety, and litigation experience in approximately 170,000 tests. *JAMA.* 1971;217(8):1061–6.
3. Irving JB, Bruce RA, DeRouen TA. Variations in and significance of systolic pressure during maximal exercise (treadmill) testing. *Am J Cardiol.* 1977;39(6):841–8.
4. McHenry PL. Risks of graded exercise testing. *Am J Cardiol.* 1977;39(6):935–7.
5. Atterhog JH, Jonsson B, Samuelsson R. Exercise testing: a prospective study of complication rates. *Am Heart J.* 1979;98(5):572–9.
6. Stuart RJ Jr, Ellestad MH. National survey of exercise stress testing facilities. *Chest.* 1980;77(1):94–7.
7. Gibbons L, Blair SN, Kohl HW, Cooper K. The safety of maximal exercise testing. *Circulation.* 1989;80(4):846–52. doi:10.1161/01.cir.80.4.846.
8. Knight JA, Laubach CA Jr, Butcher RJ, Menapace FJ. Supervision of clinical exercise testing by exercise physiologists. *Am J Cardiol.* 1995;75(5):390–1.
9. Myers J, Voodi L, Umann T, Froelicher VF. A survey of exercise testing: methods, utilization, interpretation, and safety in the VAHCS. *J Cardiopulm Rehabil.* 2000;20(4):251–8.
10. Kane GC, Hepinstall MJ, Kidd GM, et al. Safety of stress echocardiography supervised by registered nurses: results of a 2-year audit of 15,404 patients. *J Am Soc Echocardiogr.* 2008;21(4):337–41.
11. Keteyian SJ, Isaac D, Thadani U, et al. Safety of symptom-limited cardiopulmonary exercise testing in patients with chronic heart failure due to severe left ventricular systolic dysfunction. *Am Heart J.* 2009;158(4 Suppl):S72–7.
12. Skalski J, Allison TG, Miller TD. The safety of cardiopulmonary exercise testing in a population with high-risk cardiovascular diseases. *Circulation.* 2012;126(21):2465–72.

13. Rodgers GP, Ayanian JZ, Balady G, et al. American College of Cardiology/American Heart Association Clinical Competence Statement on Stress Testing. A Report of the American College of Cardiology/American Heart Association/American College of Physicians-American Society of Internal Medicine Task Force on Clinical Competence. *Circulation*. 2000;102(14):1726–38. doi:10.1161/01.cir.102.14.1726.

14. Myers J, Forman DE, Balady GJ, et al. Supervision of exercise testing by nonphysicians: a scientific statement from the American Heart Association. *Circulation*. 2014;130(12):1014–27. doi:10.1161/CIR.0000000000000101.

15. Kern KB, Halperin HR, Field J. New guidelines for cardiopulmonary resuscitation and emergency cardiac care: changes in the management of cardiac arrest. *JAMA*. 2001;285(10):1267–9. doi:10.1001/jama.285.10.1267.

16. Poole DC, Jones AM. Measurement of the maximum oxygen uptake $\dot{V}O_{2max}$: $\dot{V}O_{2peak}$ is no longer acceptable. *J Appl Physiol*. 2017;122(4):997–1002. doi:10.1152/japplphysiol.01063.2016.

17. Borg G. Psychophysical bases of perceived exertion. *Med Sci Sports Exerc*. 1982;14(5):377–81.

18. Fletcher GF, Ades PA, Kligfield P, et al. Exercise standards for testing and training: a scientific statement from the American Heart Association. *Circulation*. 2013;128(8):873–934. doi:10.1161/CIR.0b013e31829b5b44.

19. Bruce RA, Kusumi F, Hosmer D. Maximal oxygen intake and nomographic assessment of functional aerobic impairment in cardiovascular disease. *Am Heart J*. 1973;85(4):546–62. doi:10.1016/0002-8703(73)90502-4.

20. Myers J, Arena R, Franklin B, et al. Recommendations for clinical exercise laboratories: a scientific statement from the American Heart Association. *Circulation*. 2009;119(24):3144–61.

21. Balke B, Ware RW. An experimental study of physical fitness of air force personnel. *U S Armed Forces Med J*. 1959;10(6):675–88.

22. Trappe SW, Costill DL, Vukovich MD, Jones J, Melham T. Aging among elite distance runners: a 22-yr longitudinal study. *J Appl Physiol*. 1996;80(1):285–90.

23. Hansen JE, Sue DY, Wasserman K. Predicted values for clinical exercise testing. *Am Rev Respir Dis*. 1984;129(2 Pt 2):S49–55. doi:10.1164/arrd.1984.129.2P2.S49.

24. de Souza e Silva CG, Kaminsky LA, Arena R, et al. A reference equation for maximal aerobic power for treadmill and cycle ergometer exercise testing: analysis from the FRIEND Registry. *Eur J Prev Cardiol*. 2018;25(7):742–50. doi:10.1177/2047487318763958.

25. Morris CK, Myers J, Froelicher VF, et al. Nomogram based on metabolic equivalents and age for assessing aerobic exercise capacity in men. *J Am Coll Cardiol*. 1993;22(1):175–82.

26. Morris CK, Myers J, Froelicher VF, Kawaguchi T, Ueshima K, Hideg A. Nomogram based on metabolic equivalents and age for assessing aerobic exercise capacity in men. *J Am Coll Cardiol*. 1993;22(1):175–82.

27. Gulati M, Black HR, Shaw LJ, et al. The prognostic value of a nomogram for exercise capacity in women. *N Engl J Med*. 2005;353(5):468–75. doi:10.1056/NEJMoa044154.

28. Kaminsky LA, Whaley MH. Evaluation of a new standardized ramp protocol: the BSU/Bruce Ramp Protocol. *J Cardiopulm Rehabil*. 1998;18(6):438–44. doi:10.1097/00008483-199811000-00006.

29. Pollock ML, Foster C, Schmidt D, Hellman C, Linnerud AC, Ward A. Comparative analysis of physiologic responses to three different maximal graded exercise test protocols in healthy women. *Am Heart J*. 1982;103(3):363–73. doi:10.1016/0002-8703(82)90275-7.

30. Pollock ML, Bohannon RL, Cooper KH, et al. A comparative analysis of four protocols for maximal treadmill stress testing. *Am Heart J*. 1976;92(1):39–46. doi:10.1016/s0002-8703(76)80401-2.

Metabolic Calculations

CHAPTER OUTLINE

Introduction to the Use of Metabolic Calculations
- Arithmetical Reasoning for the Use of Metabolic Equations for Calculations of Physical Activity
- Expressions of Energy Use

Estimation of Energy Expenditure: The ACSM's Metabolic Calculations
- Walking Equation
- Running Equation
- Leg Ergometer Equation
- Arm Ergometer Equation
- Stepping Equation

Other Useful Equations
- Exercise Intensity Estimation Equations

Summary

Practice Problems

Answers

References

INTRODUCTION TO THE USE OF METABOLIC CALCULATIONS

As mentioned in Chapter 4, *cardiorespiratory fitness* (CRF), either via calculation or through direct measurement, refers to the integrated functional capabilities of the heart, blood vessels, lungs, and skeletal muscles to perform work. Often, exercise professionals use CRF data to (a) motivate participants to begin or maintain an exercise program, (b) individualize the exercise prescription, (c) and track progress within an exercise program. Energy requirements can be expressed in terms of the oxygen requirements of the physical activity (PA) being performed — commonly referred to as the oxygen consumption or oxygen cost ($\dot{V}O_2$). In the notation $\dot{V}O_2$,

- *V* stands for volume.
- The dot above the V ($\dot{V}$) denotes a rate, that is, the volume of oxygen consumed per unit of time — typically per minute.
- O_2 stands for oxygen.

The measure of $\dot{V}O_2$ is often used to describe maximal aerobic abilities ($\dot{V}O_{2max}$) and provides useful information for exercise professionals of their client's CRF. However, under steady-state exercise conditions, $\dot{V}O_2$ provides a measure of the energy cost of PA (frequently expressed in kilocalories) and, in combination with carbon dioxide production ($\dot{V}CO_2$), provides information about the relative mixture of metabolic substrates or fuel sources (carbohydrate vs. fat) utilized.

TABLE 6.1 • Metabolic Calculations for the Estimation of Gross Energy Expenditure (O_2 [mL · kg^{-1} · min^{-1}]) During Common Physical Activities

| | Sum of Resting + Horizontal + Vertical / Resistance Components | | | |
Mode	Resting Component	Horizontal Component	Vertical Component / Resistance Component	Limitations
Walking	3.5	0.1 × speed[a]	1.8 × speed[a] × grade[b]	Most accurate for speeds of 1.9–3.7 mph (50–100 m · min^{-1})
Running	3.5	0.2 × speed[a]	0.9 × speed[a] × grade[b]	Most accurate for speeds >5 mph (134 m · min^{-1})
Stepping	3.5	0.2 × steps · min^{-1}	1.33 × (1.8 × step height[c] × steps · min^{-1})	Most accurate for stepping rates of 12–30 steps · min^{-1}
Leg cycling	3.5	3.5	(1.8 × work rate[d]) / body mass[e]	Most accurate for work rates of 300–1200 kg · m · min^{-1} (50–200 W)
Arm cycling	3.5	—	(3 × work rate[d]) / body mass[e]	Most accurate for work rates between 150 and 750 kg · m · min^{-1} (25–125 W)

[a]Speed in m · min^{-1}.

[b]Grade is grade percentage expressed in decimal format (*e.g.*, 10% = 0.10).

[c]Step height in m.

Multiply by the following conversion factors:

lb to kg: 0.454; in to cm: 2.54; ft to m: 0.3048; mi to km: 1.609; mph to m · min^{-1}: 26.8; kg · m · min^{-1} to W: 0.164; W to kg · m · min^{-1}: 6.12; $\dot{V}O_{2max}$ L · min^{-1} to kcal · min^{-1}: 4.9; $\dot{V}O_2$ MET to mL · kg^{-1} · min^{-1}: 3.5.

[d]Work rate in kilogram-meters per minute (kg · m · min^{-1}) is calculated as resistance (kg) × distance per revolution of flywheel × pedal frequency per minute. Note: Distance per revolution is 6 m for Monark leg ergometer, 3 m for the Tunturi and BodyGuard ergometers, and 2.4 m for Monark arm ergometer.

[e]Body mass in kg.

$\dot{V}O_2$, volume of oxygen consumed per unit of time

Adapted from Swain DP, American College of Sports Medicine. *ACSM's Resource Manual for Guidelines for Exercise Testing and Prescription.* 7th ed. Philadelphia (PA): Wolters Kluwer Health/Lippincott Williams & Wilkins; 2014 (4); Whaley MH, Brubaker PH, Otto RM, Armstrong LE. *ACSM's Guidelines for Exercise Testing and Prescription.* 7th ed. Philadelphia (PA): Lippincott Williams & Wilkins; 2006 (5).

A popular method for the estimation of the energy requirements of PA employs the American College of Sports Medicine (ACSM) Metabolic Calculations (Table 6.1). This metabolic equations have been developed from regression equations derived from measured $\dot{V}O_2$ during exercise on ergometric devices and while walking and running. These equations, using basic algebra principles (*i.e.*, solving for the unknown), provide exercise professionals with a practical method to estimate the oxygen cost of common PAs (walking, running, leg cycling, arm cycling, and stepping) during steady-state, submaximal aerobic exercise.

Arithmetical Reasoning for the Use of Metabolic Equations for Calculations of Physical Activity

- Oxygen cost ($\dot{V}O_2$) for several forms of PA can be estimated.
- Oxygen cost ($\dot{V}O_2$) can be easily transferred into energy cost (kcal).
- Estimating the rate of oxygen cost during PA allows for an estimate of the energy expenditure and, hence, caloric consumption associated with the activity.
- Exercise prescription and programming can be individualized to meet a participant's needs and goals. PA programs can be individualized for a client based on their goals and needs, and precise estimates for workloads (*e.g.*, speed, grade) can be provided to achieve a certain level of metabolic stress.

Expressions of Energy Use

Energy expenditure in humans can be expressed in several ways. Converting from one expression to another is relatively simple. To better understand energy expenditure, one should be familiar with the following terms (which were mentioned in Chapters 4 and 5):

- **Aerobic metabolism:** production of energy using oxygen
- **Oxygen consumption ($\dot{V}O_2$):** expression of the amount of oxygen used or consumed
- **Absolute versus relative:** relative is an expression that involves relating the value (*e.g.*, $\dot{V}O_2$) to another value (such as body mass), whereas absolute is the expression of the value by itself.

Absolute Oxygen Consumption

This is the volume of oxygen consumed by the person per unit (minute) of time, expressed in liters per minute ($L \cdot min^{-1}$) or milliliters per minute ($mL \cdot min^{-1}$). Resting absolute oxygen consumption ($\dot{V}O_{2rest}$) for a 70-kg person is ~0.25 $L \cdot min^{-1}$. In highly trained individuals, maximal absolute oxygen consumption ($\dot{V}O_{2max}$) can be as high as 5 $L \cdot min^{-1}$.

Absolute oxygen consumption is useful because it allows for an easy estimation of caloric expenditure. Each liter of O_2 consumed by the individual is associated with an energy expenditure of ~5 kcal. This is discussed further in a later section.

Relative Oxygen Consumption

This is the oxygen consumption relative to body mass, expressed in $mL \cdot kg^{-1} \cdot min^{-1}$. In other words, it is the volume of oxygen consumed by the cells of each kilogram of body mass every minute. The resting relative oxygen consumption ($\dot{V}O_{2rest}$) is ~3.5 $mL \cdot kg^{-1} \cdot min^{-1}$. In highly trained aerobic athletes, a maximal relative oxygen consumption ($\dot{V}O_{2max}$) can be as high as 80 $mL \cdot kg^{-1} \cdot min^{-1}$. In some instances, $\dot{V}O_{2max}$ is expressed relative to a kilogram of fat-free mass, or to the square meters of body surface area, or to some other index of body size. Relative $\dot{V}O_2$ is commonly used to compare oxygen consumption of individuals who vary in body size. Because $\dot{V}O_{2max}$ is an index of CRF, a higher value is indicative of greater aerobic fitness.

An exercise professional should easily convert between absolute and relative oxygen consumption using the following formulas:

ABSOLUTE to RELATIVE

$$\frac{\dot{V}O_2 \left(L \cdot min^{-1}\right) \times 1000}{\text{Body mass (kg)}} = mL \cdot kg^{-1} \cdot min^{-1}$$

RELATIVE to ABSOLUTE

$$\frac{\dot{V}O_2 \left(mL \cdot kg^{-1} \cdot min^{-1}\right) \times \text{body mass (kg)}}{1000} = L \cdot min^{-1}$$

Example: Steve's, weighing 78 kg, absolute $\dot{V}O_{2max}$ is 2.5 $L \cdot min^{-1}$. What is his relative $\dot{V}O_{2max}$?

$$\frac{2.5 \left(L \cdot min^{-1}\right) \times 1000}{78 \text{ kg}} = 32.05 \ mL \cdot kg^{-1} \cdot min^{-1}$$

Metabolic Equivalent

A MET is an abbreviation for a metabolic equivalent. One MET is equivalent to the relative oxygen consumption at rest. Therefore, 1 MET = 3.5 $mL \cdot kg^{-1} \cdot min^{-1}$. METs are calculated by dividing the relative oxygen consumption ($mL \cdot kg^{-1} \cdot min^{-1}$) by 3.5. For example, an individual consuming 35 $mL \cdot kg^{-1} \cdot min^{-1}$ of oxygen during steady-state PA is exercising at 10 METs. A MET is a useful expression because it allows for an easy comparison of the amount of oxygen consumption during exercise with that at rest. In addition, there is not any unit of measure associated with MET(s). It is also important to point out that METs are also a useful, convenient, and standardized method for quantifying the absolute intensity of various behaviors and activities. The *2018 Physical Activity Guidelines for American* defines light-intensity PA as 1.6 to 2.9 METs, moderate as 3 to 5.9 METs, and vigorous as ≥6 METs (1). Lastly, MET can also be converted to caloric expenditure (which is discussed in the next section).

$$1 \text{ MET} = 1 \text{ kcal} \cdot hr^{-1} \cdot kg^{-1}$$

Calories

This expression of energy intake and expenditure is commonly used to quantify the amount of energy derived from foodstuffs as well as the amount of energy expended at rest and during PA. A calorie is a very small unit. Most often, kilocalories (kcal) is used. One kilocalorie equals 1000 calories. An average-sized individual who runs or walks 1 mi expends ~100 kcal. Also, a somewhat useful comparison for weight management is that every pound of fat contains about 3500 kcal. When disregarding the respiratory exchange ratio (RER), which is discussed in a later section, the ratio between oxygen consumption and energy expenditure is 5 kcal for every liter of oxygen consumed ($5 \ kcal \cdot L^{-1}$). The kilocalorie can also be expressed in terms of a rate ($kcal \cdot min^{-1}$) and is then very useful in terms of the absolute energy intensity of exercise. For instance, one can express the exercise intensity in terms of $kcal \cdot min^{-1}$. An exercise of $10 \ kcal \cdot min^{-1}$ means the individual is expending 10 kcal of energy for every minute they exercise:

$$10 \ kcal \cdot min^{-1} = \frac{10 \ kcal \cdot min^{-1}}{5 \ kcal \cdot L^{-1}} = 2 \ L \cdot min^{-1} \ oxygen \ consumption$$

Respiratory Exchange Ratio

The RER may be used to assess the relative use of carbohydrates versus fats in aerobic metabolism (assuming that the amino acids from proteins are not a major supplier of ATP for exercise catabolism). The RER is the ratio of the carbon dioxide produced and the oxygen consumed ($RER = \dot{V}CO_2 / \dot{V}O_2$). When the RER is close to 0.70, fats are the primary fuel source for energy metabolism. When the RER is closer to 1, the primary fuel source for energy metabolism is carbohydrates. When the RER is given or can be calculated, $\dot{V}CO_2 / \dot{V}O_2$, the ratio between oxygen consumption and energy expenditure, is $~4.0 + RER$ kcal for every liter of oxygen consumed. For example, if the RER for a given activity is 0.85, the energy expenditure would be 4.85 kcal for every liter of oxygen consumed ($4.85 \ kcal \cdot L^{-1}$).

Carbohydrate and Fat Stores   Carbohydrates are stored in three main areas in the body: (a) in skeletal muscle as glycogen, (b) in the liver as glycogen, and (c) in the blood as glucose. For an individual weighing 65 kg, the total storage of carbohydrates in the body may be ~2500 kcal (2). The human body stores the majority of excess energy intake as fat stored either below the skin (subcutaneous fat) or around the internal organs (visceral fat) with limited amounts intramuscularly. The amount of fat one stores for energy usage can be represented by one's body composition, or percent body fat. The same 65-kg individual stores ~75,000 kcal of fat. It takes ~3500 calories to make and store 1 lb of body fat. Stated in reverse, 1 lb of fat can provide the body with 3500 calories — the amount of energy needed to walk or run about 35 mi!

Net Versus Gross $\dot{V}O_2$

Gross $\dot{V}O_2$ refers to the total oxygen consumption, whereas net $\dot{V}O_2$ refers to the oxygen consumption for only the activity portion (or minus the resting component). All ACSM's Metabolic Calculations provide gross $\dot{V}O_2$ values. In terms of exercise prescription, it may be helpful to use the net $\dot{V}O_2$ value (thus you may need to delete the resting component) ($3.5 \ mL \cdot kg^{-1} \cdot min^{-1}$).

Net $\dot{V}O_2$ may also be used to assess the caloric cost of exercise. Net and gross oxygen consumption can be expressed in relative or absolute terms. The net $\dot{V}O_2$ is calculated by subtracting the resting $\dot{V}O_2$ from the gross $\dot{V}O_2$:

$$Net \ \dot{V}O_2 = Gross \ \dot{V}O_2 - resting \ \dot{V}O_2$$

- The gross rate of oxygen consumption is the total $\dot{V}O_2$ including the resting oxygen required, expressed as either $L \cdot min^{-1}$ or $3.5 \ mL \cdot kg^{-1} \cdot min^{-1}$.
- The net rate of oxygen consumption is the $\dot{V}O_2$ associated with only the amount of exercise being performed exclusive of resting oxygen uptake, expressed as either $L \cdot min^{-1}$ or $3.5 \ mL \cdot kg^{-1} \cdot min^{-1}$.

ESTIMATION OF ENERGY EXPENDITURE: THE ACSM'S METABOLIC CALCULATIONS

In Table 6.1, there are five metabolic equations: walking, running, leg ergometry, arm ergometry, and stepping. A few important conditions concerning these equations to note are as follows:

- All metabolic equations are expressed in $mL \cdot kg^{-1} \cdot min^{-1}$ (relative terms).
- All metabolic equations are estimated gross or total energy cost.

- When using these equations to determine caloric expenditure, one should use **net** $\dot{V}O_2$ by subtracting the resting $\dot{V}O_2$, 3.5 mL $\cdot$ kg^{-1} $\cdot$ min^{-1} or 1 MET.
- The measured $\dot{V}O_2$ at a given work rate is highly reproducible for a given individual; that is, the $\dot{V}O_2$ at the same exercise intensity for the same individual will be very similar every time they exercise. However, the intersubject variability (variability between different subjects) in measured $\dot{V}O_2$ may have a standard error of estimate (SEE) as high as 7%.
- These equations were derived during steady-state submaximal aerobic exercise; therefore, they are only appropriate for predicting $\dot{V}O_2$ during steady-state submaximal aerobic exercise. The $\dot{V}O_2$ will be overestimated or underestimated when the contribution from anaerobic metabolism is large (such as near-maximal exertion) or during non–steady-state exercise conditions.
  - When using the ACSM's metabolic equations, be sure that the exercise being conducted is both submaximal and steady state.
- Although the accuracy of these equations is unaffected by most environmental influences (*e.g.*, heat and cold), variables that change the mechanical efficiency (*e.g.*, gait abnormalities, wind, snow, or sand) will result in a loss of accuracy.
- The use of the ACSM's metabolic equations presupposes that ergometers are calibrated properly and used appropriately (*e.g.*, no rail holding during treadmill exercise).
- The equations are most accurate at the stated speeds and power outputs (see Table 6.1, right column).

Walking Equation

The ACSM's walking equation is a useful tool for determining proper training intensity and also can be used to estimate caloric expenditure during walking activities.

Derivation of the Walking Equation

There are three components within the walking equation, each representing an aspect of energy expenditure, horizontal, vertical, and resting components.

The oxygen cost of moving 1 kg of body weight 1 m has been estimated to be 0.1 mL $\cdot$ kg^{-1} $\cdot$ min^{-1}. Therefore, the horizontal component of walking can be computed as follows:

$$\textbf{Horizontal component} = \text{Speed (m} \cdot \text{min}^{-1}) \times 0.1 \text{ mL} \cdot \text{kg}^{-1} \cdot \text{min}^{-1}$$

- Note that treadmill speed in miles per hour (mph) **must** be converted to m $\cdot$ min^{-1} to be used in the walking equation. The conversion factor is 1 mph = 26.8 m $\cdot$ min^{-1}.
  - Example: What would be the speed in m $\cdot$ min^{-1} of walking at 2.5 mph?

$$2.5 \text{ mph} \times 26.8 \text{ m} \cdot \text{min}^{-1} = 67 \text{ m} \cdot \text{min}^{-1}$$

The vertical component of walking can be calculated if we know the oxygen cost of moving vertically against gravity. This has been estimated to be 1.8 mL $\cdot$ min^{-1} for each meter walked. Since the rate of movement (speed) as well as the steepness of the vertical climb (grade) also must be known, the vertical component contains all three of these components.

$$\textbf{Vertical component} = \text{Speed (m} \cdot \text{min}^{-1}) \times \text{Grade (decimal)} \times 1.8 \text{ mL} \cdot \text{kg}^{-1} \cdot \text{min}^{-1}$$

Computing Grade

Vertical ascent is denoted by grade, typically computed as a fraction (decimal) and then converted to a percent. Percent grade reflects the degree of elevation gain for a given horizontal distance.

Example: A rise of 1 foot over a distance of 10 ft?

$$= 1 \text{ ft} / 10 \text{ ft} = 0.10 \qquad 0.10 \times 100 = 10\% \text{ grade}$$

Note that when expressing grade within the walking equation, it is done in <u>decimal form</u>:

$$\text{Example: } 10\% \text{ grade} = \textbf{0.10} \qquad 5\% \text{ grade} = \textbf{0.05}$$

Together, the horizontal and vertical components represent the net O_2 cost of walking; meaning the O_2 cost above rest. To obtain the gross $\dot{V}O_2$, we must add in the O_2 cost at rest (3.5 mL $\cdot$ kg^{-1} $\cdot$ min^{-1}). Resting metabolic rate has been computed at 1 MET, or 3.5 mL $\cdot$ kg^{-1} $\cdot$ min^{-1}. This value is added in at the end of the equation and is known as the *resting component*.

$$\textbf{Resting component} = 3.5 \text{ mL} \cdot \text{kg}^{-1} \cdot \text{min}^{-1}$$

The ACSM's Walking Equation

$$\dot{V}O_2 \text{ mL} \cdot \text{kg}^{-1} \cdot \text{min}^{-1} = [\text{Speed (m} \cdot \text{min}^{-1}) \times 0.1 \text{ mL} \cdot \text{kg}^{-1} \cdot \text{min}^{-1}] + [\text{Speed (m} \cdot \text{min}^{-1})$$
$$\times \text{ Grade (decimal)} \times 1.8 \text{ mL} \cdot \text{kg}^{-1} \cdot \text{min}^{-1}] + 3.5 \text{ mL} \cdot \text{kg}^{-1} \cdot \text{min}^{-1}$$

Limitations of the Walking Equation

1. Steady-State Exercise Only!
    1. The ACSM's walking equation was computed based on steady-state oxygen consumption values. Therefore, the equation will not be accurate when computing oxygen consumption during non–steady-state exercise. Using the ACSM's walking equation to compute a maximal oxygen uptake (*e.g.*, the last stage of a maximal exercise test) will not be accurate during such non–steady-state exercise.
2. Accuracy is dependent on speed range!
    1. The ACSM's walking equation is only accurate between 1.9 (46 m·min^{-1}) and 3.7 (100 m·min^{-1}) miles per hour.. Above the given speed range, walking economy changes, and individuals of differing height may actually run.

Examples and Solutions for the Walking Equation

1. Bob walks at 3.2 mph up a 3% incline. Calculate Bob's oxygen cost.
    - $\dot{V}O_2 \text{ mL} \cdot \text{kg}^{-1} \cdot \text{min}^{-1} = [S \text{ (m} \cdot \text{min}^{-1}) \times 0.1] + [S \text{ (m} \cdot \text{min}^{-1}) \times G \text{ (dec)} \times 1.8] + 3.5$
        - Speed (S) conversion: 3.2 mph $\times$ 26.8 = 85.76 m $\cdot$ min^{-1}
        - Grade (G) conversion: 3% / 100 = 0.03
    - $\dot{V}O_2 \text{ mL} \cdot \text{kg}^{-1} \cdot \text{min}^{-1} = [85.76 \times 0.1] + [85.76 \times 0.03 \times 1.8] + 3.5$
    - $\dot{V}O_2 \text{ mL} \cdot \text{kg}^{-1} \cdot \text{min}^{-1} = 8.58 + 4.63 + 3.5 = \textbf{16.71 mL} \cdot \textbf{kg}^{-1} \cdot \textbf{min}^{-1}$
2. You are prescribing a walking exercise to your participant Jane and you would like her to walk at 10.75 mL $\cdot$ kg^{-1} $\cdot$ min^{-1} oxygen cost with no incline (grade is 0%). Calculate Jane's walking speed in mph.
    - $\dot{V}O_2 \text{ mL} \cdot \text{kg}^{-1} \cdot \text{min}^{-1} = [S \text{ (m} \cdot \text{min}^{-1}) \times 0.1] + [S \text{ (m} \cdot \text{min}^{-1}) \times G \text{ (dec)} \times 1.8] + 3.5$
    - $10.75 = [S \text{ (m} \cdot \text{min}^{-1}) \times 0.10] + [S \cdot \text{m} \cdot \text{min}^{-1} \times 0 \times 1.8] + 3.5$
    - Subtract 3.5 from both sides of the equation
        - $7.25 = [\ S \text{ (m} \cdot \text{min}^{-1}) \times 0.10] + 0$
    - Divide both sides by 0.10
        - $\dfrac{7.25}{0.10} = [S \text{ (m} \cdot \text{min}^{-1}) \times \dfrac{0.10}{0.10}] = \textbf{72.5 m} \cdot \textbf{min}^{-1}$
    - $\dfrac{72.5 \text{ m} \cdot \text{min}^{-1}}{26.8} = \textbf{2.7 mph}$
3. Steve typically jogs at a pace equivalent to a $\dot{V}O_2$ of 30 mL $\cdot$ kg^{-1} $\cdot$ min^{-1}. Due to an injury, you wish to have Steve walk at 3.5 mph, yet walk on an incline that will elicit the same $\dot{V}O_2$ (30 mL $\cdot$ kg^{-1} $\cdot$ min^{-1}). What is the appropriate grade?
    - $\dot{V}O_2 \text{ mL} \cdot \text{kg}^{-1} \cdot \text{min}^{-1} = [S \text{ (m} \cdot \text{min}^{-1}) \times 0.1] + [S \text{ (m} \cdot \text{min}^{-1}) \times G \text{ (dec)} \times 1.8] + 3.5$
        - Speed (S) conversion: 3.5 mph $\times$ 26.8 = 93.8 m $\cdot$ min^{-1}
    - $30 \text{ mL} \cdot \text{kg}^{-1} \cdot \text{min}^{-1} = [93.8 \times 0.10] + [93.8 \times G \times 1.8] + 3.5$
    - Subtract 3.5 from both sides of the equation
        - $26.5 = 9.38 + 168.84 \times G$
    - Subtract 9.38 from both sides of the equation
        - $17.12 = 168.84 \times G$

- Divide both sides by 168.84
  - $\dfrac{17.12}{168.84} = \dfrac{168.84\,G}{168.84}$
- 0.1
- **$G = 0.1 \times 100 = 10\%$**

Running Equation

Similar to the ACSM's walking equation, the ACSM's running equation is a useful tool for determining proper training intensity as well as estimating caloric expenditure during running activities.

Derivation of the Running Equation

As the case with the walking equation, the running equation is also composed of three components: horizontal, vertical, and resting.

The horizontal component of the running equation requires twice the oxygen compared to horizontal walking. Thus, the horizontal component is computed as:

$$\textbf{Horizontal component} = \text{Speed (m} \cdot \text{min}^{-1}) \times 0.2 \text{ mL} \cdot \text{kg}^{-1} \cdot \text{min}^{-1}$$

- Remember to convert to m · min^{-1}

The vertical component does not have the same oxygen cost for running as it does for walking. The vertical component can be computed as:

$$\textbf{Vertical component} = \text{Speed (m} \cdot \text{min}^{-1}) \times \text{Grade (decimal)} \times 0.9 \text{ mL} \cdot \text{kg}^{-1} \cdot \text{min}^{-1}$$

- Remember to compute the grade

$$\textbf{Resting component} = 3.5 \text{ mL} \cdot \text{kg}^{-1} \cdot \text{min}^{-1}$$

The ACSM'S Running Equation

$$\dot{V}O_2 \text{ mL} \cdot \text{kg}^{-1} \cdot \text{min}^{-1} = [\text{Speed (m} \cdot \text{min}^{-1}) \times 0.2 \text{ mL} \cdot \text{kg}^{-1} \cdot \text{min}^{-1}] + [\text{Speed (m} \cdot \text{min}^{-1})$$
$$\times \text{ Grade (decimal)} \times 0.9 \text{ mL} \cdot \text{kg}^{-1} \cdot \text{min}^{-1}] + 3.5 \text{ mL} \cdot \text{kg}^{-1} \cdot \text{min}^{-1}$$

Limitations of the Running Equation

1. Steady-state exercise only!
   1. Similar to the ACSM's walking equation, the ACSM's running equation was computed based on steady-state oxygen consumption values. Therefore, the equation will not be accurate when computing oxygen consumption during non–steady-state exercise.

Accuracy is dependent on speed range!

2. Generally, the running equation is designed for speeds greater than 5 mph (134 m · min^{-1}). However, depending on body size and preference, some individuals may choose to run at speeds as low as 3.7 mph (100 m · min^{-1}). Individual analysis will determine which equation (walk or run) should be used. For example, if the client is jogging at 4 mph, then it would be appropriate to use the running equation.

Examples and Solutions for the Running Equation

1. John is jogging at 5.6 mph up a 2.5% incline. What is the oxygen cost?
   - $\dot{V}O_2$ mL · kg^{-1} · min^{-1} = [S (m · min^{-1}) × 0.2] + [S (m · min^{-1}) × G (dec) × 0.9] + 3.5
     - Speed (S) conversion: 5.6 mph × 26.8 = 150.08 m · min^{-1}
     - Grade (G) conversion: 2.5% / 100 = 0.025
   - $\dot{V}O_2$ mL · kg^{-1} · min^{-1} = [150.08 × 0.2] + [150.08 × 0.025 × 0.9] + 3.5
   - $\dot{V}O_2$ mL · kg^{-1} · min^{-1} = 30.02 + 3.38 + 3.5 = **36.90 mL · kg^{-1} · min^{-1}**
2. You are prescribing a running exercise to your participant; George would like to run at 39 mL · kg^{-1} · min^{-1} oxygen cost with a 2% incline. Calculate George's running speed in mph.
   - $\dot{V}O_2$ mL · kg^{-1} · min^{-1} = [S (m · min^{-1}) × 0.2] + [S (m · min^{-1}) × G (dec) × 0.9] + 3.5

- $39 \text{ mL} \cdot \text{kg}^{-1} \cdot \text{min}^{-1} = [S \,(\text{m} \cdot \text{min}^{-1}) \times 0.2] + [S \,(\text{m} \cdot \text{min}^{-1}) \times 0.02 \times 0.9] + 3.5$
- Subtract 3.5 from both sides of the equation
  - $35.5 = [S \,(\text{m} \cdot \text{min}^{-1}) \times 0.20] + [S \,(\text{m} \cdot \text{min}^{-1}) \times 0.018]$
  - $35.5 = [S \,(\text{m} \cdot \text{min}^{-1}) \times 0.218]$
- Divide both sides by 0.22
  - $\dfrac{35.5}{0.22} = \left[S \,(\text{m} \cdot \text{min}^{-1}) \times \dfrac{0.10}{0.10}\right] = \mathbf{161.36 \text{ m} \cdot \text{min}^{-1}}$
- $\dfrac{161.36 \text{ m} \cdot \text{min}^{-1}}{26.8} = \mathbf{6 \text{ mph}}$

3. Jay has been an avid exerciser for a while, and his preferred intensity is equivalent to $45 \text{ mL} \cdot \text{kg}^{-1} \cdot \text{min}^{-1}$. Jay would like to run at 5.5 mph. What is the appropriate treadmill incline to achieve $45 \text{ mL} \cdot \text{kg}^{-1} \cdot \text{min}^{-1}$?
   - $\dot{V}O_2 \text{ mL} \cdot \text{kg}^{-1} \cdot \text{min}^{-1} = [S \,(\text{m} \cdot \text{min}^{-1}) \times 0.2] + [S \,(\text{m} \cdot \text{min}^{-1}) \times G \,(\text{dec}) \times 0.9] + 3.5$
     - Speed (S) conversion: $5.5 \text{ mph} \times 26.8 = 147.4 \text{ m} \cdot \text{min}^{-1}$
   - $45 \text{ mL} \cdot \text{kg}^{-1} \cdot \text{min}^{-1} = [147.4 \times 0.20] + [147.4 \times G \times 0.9] + 3.5$
   - Subtract 3.5 from both sides of the equation
     - $41.5 = 29.48 + 132.66 \times G$
   - Subtract 29.48 from both sides of the equation.
     - $12.02 = 132.66 \times G$
   - Divide both sides by 132.66
     - $\dfrac{12.02}{132.66} = \dfrac{132.66 \, G}{132.66}$
   - $\mathbf{0.09}$
   - $\mathbf{G = 0.09 \times 100 = 9\%}$

Leg Ergometer Equation

The leg ergometer, or cycle ergometer, as it is commonly called, is one of the most common modes of both testing and exercise. Leg ergometers are commonly used for submaximal exercise testing and aerobic training in a health fitness setting.

Derivation of the Leg Ergometer Equation

During leg ergometer exercise, the client is pedaling against a resistance, which moves a flywheel a given distance with each turn of the pedal crank. Computing the number of pedal turns in a minute helps us compute the work rate. Work rate during leg ergometer exercise is computed in kilogram-meters per minute ($\text{kg} \cdot \text{m} \cdot \text{min}^{-1}$):

$$\text{Work rate } (\text{kg} \cdot \text{m} \cdot \text{min}^{-1}) = R \,(\text{kg}) \times D \,(\text{m}) \times \text{rev} \cdot \text{min}^{-1}$$

where R = resistance or gravitational force, expressed as kilogram-force (kg)
D = distance in meters the flywheel travels with each pedal crank
$\text{rev} \cdot \text{min}^{-1}$ = revolutions (pedal cranks) per minute

- Note and as mentioned in Chapter 4, we are using the resistance as kilogram-force (kg), it is also common to see gravitational force expressed as kilopond (kp), from Latin in which *pondus* means weight.
- Note that the flywheel on a leg ergometer may vary by manufacturer. Therefore, depending on the ergometer manufacturer, the distance the flywheel travels with each pedal revolution will vary by manufacturer:
  - Monark leg ergometers: 6 m per pedal revolution
  - Tunturi leg ergometers: 3 m per pedal revolution
  - Be sure to identify the type of leg ergometer being used, so that you can accurately quantify work rate.

- Note that work rate can also be expressed in watts. These units are commonly used in health and fitness settings as well as in the research literature. Conversion from $kg \cdot m \cdot min^{-1}$ to watts is quite simple:

$$\text{Watts} = \frac{kg \cdot m \cdot min^{-1}}{6.12} \text{ or } kg \cdot m \cdot min^{-1} = \text{watts} \times 6.12$$

There are three components within the leg ergometer equation, each representing an aspect of energy expenditure, unloaded cycling, resistance, and resting components.

The oxygen cost of simply moving the flywheel as well as the movement of the legs themselves is ~3.5 $mL \cdot kg^{-1} \cdot min^{-1}$ and is defined as horizontal/unloaded cycling. This applies to pedal revolutions of 50 to 60 $rev \cdot min^{-1}$, so the cost may vary when pedaling outside this range.

Unloaded cycling component = 3.5 $mL \cdot kg^{-1} \cdot min^{-1}$

The external resistance or load placed on the flywheel is ~1.8 $mL \cdot kg^{-1} \cdot min^{-1}$ for each $kg \cdot m \cdot min^{-1}$ per body mass in kg.

$$\textbf{Vertical component} = \frac{1.8 \ mL \cdot kg^{-1} \cdot min^{-1} \times \text{work rate } (kg \cdot m \cdot min^{-1})}{\text{body mass (kg)}}$$

Resting component = 3.5 $mL \cdot kg^{-1} \cdot min^{-1}$

The ACSM's Leg Ergometer Equation

$$\dot{V}O_2 \ mL \cdot kg^{-1} \cdot min^{-1} = [1.8 \ mL \cdot kg^{-1} \cdot min^{-1} \times \frac{\text{work rate } (kg \cdot m \cdot min^{-1})}{\text{body mass (kg)}}] + 3.5 \ mL \cdot kg^{-1} \cdot min^{-1} + 3.5 \ mL \cdot kg^{-1} \cdot min^{-1}$$

Can be expressed more simply:

$$\dot{V}O_2 \ mL \cdot kg^{-1} \cdot min^{-1} = [1.8 \ mL \cdot kg^{-1} \cdot min^{-1} \times \frac{\text{work rate } (kg \cdot m \cdot min^{-1})}{\text{body mass (kg)}}] + 7 \ mL \cdot kg^{-1} \cdot min^{-1}$$

Limitations of the Leg Ergometer Equation

1. Steady-State Exercise Only!
   1. The ACSM's leg ergometer equation was computed based on steady-state oxygen consumption values. Therefore, the equation will not be as accurate when computing oxygen consumption during non–steady-state exercise. Using the ACSM's leg ergometer equation to compute a maximal oxygen uptake (*e.g.*, the last stage of a maximal exercise test) will not be accurate during such non–steady-state exercise.
2. Work rates from 300 to 1200 $kg \cdot m \cdot min^{-1}$
   1. In watts, the accuracy is between ~50 and 200. Fit individuals may exercise beyond these work rates, so the potential error increases as work rates exceed this range.

Examples and Solutions for the Leg Ergometer Equation

1. Bob, weighing 90.91 kg, cycles on a Monark leg ergometer at 50 $rev \cdot min^{-1}$ against 2 kg resistance. Calculate Bob's oxygen cost.
   - $\dot{V}O_2 \ mL \cdot kg^{-1} \cdot min^{-1} = [1.8 \ mL \cdot kg^{-1} \cdot min^{-1} \times \frac{\text{work rate } (kg \cdot m \cdot min^{-1})}{\text{body mass (kg)}}] + 7 \ mL \cdot kg^{-1} \cdot min^{-1}$
      - Work rate = $(kg \cdot m \cdot min^{-1}) = R \ (kg) \times D \ (m) \times rev \cdot min^{-1}$
      - Work rate = $(kg \cdot m \cdot min^{-1}) = 2 \ kg \times 6 \ m \times 50 \ rev \cdot min^{-1} = 600 \ kg \cdot m \cdot min^{-1}$
   - $\dot{V}O_2 \ mL \cdot kg^{-1} \cdot min^{-1} = [1.8 \ mL \cdot kg^{-1} \cdot min^{-1} \times \frac{600 \ kg \cdot m \cdot min^{-1}}{90.91 \ kg}] + 7 \ mL \cdot kg^{-1} \cdot min^{-1}$
   - $\dot{V}O_2 \ mL \cdot kg^{-1} \cdot min^{-1} = 11.88 + 7 = \textbf{18.88 mL} \cdot \textbf{kg}^{-1} \cdot \textbf{min}^{-1}$

2. Robert, weighing 75 kg, cycles on a Monark leg ergometer. If his oxygen cost is 19.96 mL $\cdot$ kg$^{-1} \cdot$ min^{-1}, what is his work rate?

- $\dot{V}O_2$ mL $\cdot$ kg$^{-1} \cdot$ min^{-1} = $\left[1.8 \text{ mL} \cdot \text{kg}^{-1} \cdot \text{min}^{-1} \times \dfrac{\text{work rate (kg} \cdot \text{m} \cdot \text{min}^{-1})}{\text{body mass (kg)}} \right]$ + 7 mL $\cdot$ kg$^{-1} \cdot$ min^{-1}

- 19.96 mL $\cdot$ kg$^{-1} \cdot$ min^{-1} = $\left[1.8 \text{ mL} \cdot \text{kg}^{-1} \cdot \text{min}^{-1} \times \dfrac{\text{work rate (kg} \cdot \text{m} \cdot \text{min}^{-1})}{75 \text{ kg}} \right]$ + 7 mL $\cdot$ kg$^{-1} \cdot$ min^{-1}

- Subtract 7 from both sides of the equation

  - 12.96 mL $\cdot$ kg$^{-1} \cdot$ min^{-1} = $\left[1.8 \text{ mL} \cdot \text{kg}^{-1} \cdot \text{min}^{-1} \times \dfrac{\text{work rate (kg} \cdot \text{m} \cdot \text{min}^{-1})}{75 \text{ kg}} \right]$ 7 mL $\cdot$ kg$^{-1} \cdot$ min^{-1}

- Multiply both sides by 75
  - 972 = 1.8 work rate
- Divide both sides by 1.8
  - Work rate = $\dfrac{972}{1.8}$ = **540 kg $\cdot$ m $\cdot$ min^{-1}**

3. Julia, weighing 50 kg, cycles on a Monark leg ergometer. Assuming that oxygen cost for the exercise is 22 mL $\cdot$ kg$^{-1} \cdot$ min^{-1}, calculate her work rate in watts?

- $\dot{V}O_2$ mL $\cdot$ kg$^{-1} \cdot$ min^{-1} = $[1.8 \text{ mL} \cdot \text{kg}^{-1} \cdot \text{min}^{-1} \times \dfrac{\text{work rate (kg} \cdot \text{m} \cdot \text{min}^{-1})}{\text{body mass (kg)}}]$ + 7 mL $\cdot$ kg$^{-1} \cdot$ min^{-1}

- 22 mL $\cdot$ kg$^{-1} \cdot$ min^{-1} = $[1.8 \text{ mL} \cdot \text{kg}^{-1} \cdot \text{min}^{-1} \times \dfrac{\text{work rate (kg} \cdot \text{m} \cdot \text{min}^{-1})}{50 \text{ kg}}]$ + 7 mL $\cdot$ kg$^{-1} \cdot$ min^{-1}
- Subtract 7 from both sides of the equation

  - 15 mL $\cdot$ kg$^{-1} \cdot$ min^{-1} = $[1.8 \text{ mL} \cdot \text{kg}^{-1} \cdot \text{min}^{-1} \times \dfrac{\text{work rate (kg} \cdot \text{m} \cdot \text{min}^{-1})}{50 \text{ kg}}]$

- Multiply both sides by 50
  - 750 = 1.8 work rate
- Divide both sides by 1.8

  - Work rate = $\dfrac{750}{1.8}$ = 417 kg $\cdot$ m $\cdot$ min^{-1}

- Convert to watts

  - Work rate = $\dfrac{\text{kg} \cdot \text{m} \cdot \text{min}^{-1}}{6.12}$ = $\dfrac{417 \text{ kg} \cdot \text{m} \cdot \text{min}^{-1}}{6.12}$ = **68.13** W

Arm Ergometer Equation

The arm ergometer is a useful device for both exercise testing and training. In cases where an individual is unable to perform lower body exercise, or when you wish to determine arm-specific aerobic power, the arm ergometer is used. Be aware that during arm exercise, owing to the reduced muscle mass involved, blood pressure will be higher at a given heart rate (HR) than during lower body exercise. In addition, work rates assigned will be much lower than leg ergometer exercise.

Derivation of the Arm Ergometer Equation

In arm ergometer exercise, the client is pedaling against a resistance, which moves a flywheel a given distance with each turn of the pedal crank. Computing the number of pedal turns in a minute helps us compute the work rate. Similar to the leg ergometer, work rate during arm ergometer exercise is computed in kilogram-meters per minute (kg $\cdot$ m $\cdot$ min^{-1}) and using the same equation.

- Note and as mentioned in Chapter 4, in this text we are using the resistance as kilogram-force (kg), it is also common to see gravitational force expressed as kilopond (kp), from Latin in which *pondus* means weight.
- Note that the flywheel on the arm ergometer may vary by manufacturer; however, the Monark arm ergometer is commonly used. This will be the ergometer that examples will be based on. Monark arm ergometers have a flywheel that moves 2.4 m per pedal revolution.

● Similar to the leg ergometer, work rate can also be expressed in watts:

$$\text{Watts} = \frac{\text{kg} \cdot \text{m} \cdot \text{min}^{-1}}{6.12} \text{ or kg} \cdot \text{m} \cdot \text{min}^{-1} = \text{watts} \times 6.12$$

Similar to leg ergometer, there are three components within the arm ergometer equation, each representing an aspect of energy expenditure, unloaded cycling (negligible), resistance, and resting components.

The oxygen cost of unloaded arm cycling is negligible and, therefore, not included in the equation.

Unloaded arm cycling component $= 0 \text{ mL} \cdot \text{kg}^{-1} \cdot \text{min}^{-1}$

The external resistance or load placed on the flywheel is ~3 mL · kg^{-1} · min^{-1} for each kg · m · min^{-1} per body mass in kilogram.

Vertical component $= \dfrac{3 \text{ mL} \cdot \text{kg}^{-1} \cdot \text{min}^{-1} \times \text{work rate (kg} \cdot \text{m} \cdot \text{min}^{-1})}{\text{body mass (kg)}}$

Resting component $= 3.5 \text{ mL} \cdot \text{kg}^{-1} \cdot \text{min}^{-1}$

The ACSM's Arm Ergometer Equation

$$\dot{V}O_2 \text{ mL} \cdot \text{kg}^{-1} \cdot \text{min}^{-1} = [3 \text{ mL} \cdot \text{kg}^{-1} \cdot \text{min}^{-1} \times \frac{\text{work rate (kg} \cdot \text{m} \cdot \text{min}^{-1})}{\text{body mass (kg)}}] + 3.5 \text{ mL} \cdot \text{kg}^{-1} \cdot \text{min}^{-1}$$

Limitations of the Arm Ergometer Equation

1. Steady-State Exercise Only!
   1. The ACSM's arm ergometer equation was computed based on steady-state oxygen consumption values. Therefore, the equation will not be as accurate when computing oxygen consumption during non–steady-state exercise.
2. Work rates from 150 to 750 kg · m · min^{-1}
   1. In watts, the accuracy is between ~25 and 125. Fit individuals may exercise beyond these work rates, so the potential error increases as work rates exceed this range.

Examples and Solutions for the Arm Ergometer Equation

1. Bob, weighing 90.91 kg, cycles on a Monark arm ergometer at 50 rev · min^{-1} against 1 kg resistance. Calculate Bob's work rate.
   ● Work rate $= (\text{kg} \cdot \text{m} \cdot \text{min}^{-1}) = R \text{ (kg)} \times D \text{ (m)} \times \text{rev} \cdot \text{min}^{-1}$
   ● Work rate $= (\text{kg} \cdot \text{m} \cdot \text{min}^{-1}) = 1 \text{ kg} \times 2.4 \text{ m} \times 50 \text{ rev} \cdot \text{min}^{-1} = \mathbf{120 \text{ kg} \cdot \text{m} \cdot \text{min}^{-1}}$
2. Amy, weighing 50 kg, trains on a Monark arm ergometer. If her oxygen cost is 10 mL · kg^{-1} · min^{-1}, what is her work rate?
   ● $\dot{V}O_2 \text{ mL} \cdot \text{kg}^{-1} \cdot \text{min}^{-1} = [3 \text{ mL} \cdot \text{kg}^{-1} \cdot \text{min}^{-1} \times \dfrac{\text{work rate (kg} \cdot \text{m} \cdot \text{min}^{-1})}{\text{body mass (kg)}}] + 3.5 \text{ mL} \cdot \text{kg}^{-1} \cdot \text{min}^{-1}$

   ● $10 \text{ mL} \cdot \text{kg}^{-1} \cdot \text{min}^{-1} = [3 \text{ mL} \cdot \text{kg}^{-1} \cdot \text{min}^{-1} \times \dfrac{\text{work rate (kg} \cdot \text{m} \cdot \text{min}^{-1})}{50 \text{ kg}}] + 3.5 \text{ mL} \cdot \text{kg}^{-1} \cdot \text{min}^{-1}$
   ● Subtract 3.5 from both sides of the equation

   ● $6.5 \text{ mL} \cdot \text{kg}^{-1} \cdot \text{min}^{-1} = \left[3 \text{ mL} \cdot \text{kg}^{-1} \cdot \text{min}^{-1} \times \dfrac{\text{work rate (kg} \cdot \text{m} \cdot \text{min}^{-1})}{50 \text{ kg}}\right]$
   ● Multiply both sides by 50
      ● $325 = 3 \text{ work rate}$
   ● Divide both sides by 3
      ● Work rate $= \dfrac{325}{3} = \mathbf{108.33 \text{ kg} \cdot \text{m} \cdot \text{min}^{-1}}$

3. Jalen, weighing 95 kg, cycles on a Monark arm ergometer. Assuming that oxygen cost for the exercise is 25 mL · kg^{-1} · min^{-1}, calculate his work rate in watts?
   ● $\dot{V}O_2 \text{ mL} \cdot \text{kg}^{-1} \cdot \text{min}^{-1} = [3 \text{ mL} \cdot \text{kg}^{-1} \cdot \text{min}^{-1} \times \dfrac{\text{work rate (kg} \cdot \text{m} \cdot \text{min}^{-1})}{\text{body mass (kg)}}] + 3.5 \text{ mL} \cdot \text{kg}^{-1} \cdot \text{min}^{-1}$
   ● $25 \text{ mL} \cdot \text{kg}^{-1} \cdot \text{min}^{-1} = [3 \text{ mL} \cdot \text{kg}^{-1} \cdot \text{min}^{-1} \times \dfrac{\text{work rate (kg} \cdot \text{m} \cdot \text{min}^{-1})}{95 \text{ kg}}] + 3.5 \text{ mL} \cdot \text{kg}^{-1} \cdot \text{min}^{-1}$

- Subtract 3.5 from both sides of the equation
  - $21.5 \text{ mL} \cdot \text{kg}^{-1} \cdot \text{min}^{-1} = [3 \text{ mL} \cdot \text{kg}^{-1} \cdot \text{min}^{-1} \times \dfrac{\text{work rate (kg} \cdot \text{m} \cdot \text{min}^{-1})}{95 \text{ kg}}]$
- Multiply both sides by 95
  - $2043 = 3 \text{ work rate}$
- Divide both sides by 3
  - $\text{Work rate} = \dfrac{2043}{3} = 681 \text{ kg} \cdot \text{m} \cdot \text{min}^{-1}$
- Convert to watts
  - $\text{Watts} = \dfrac{\text{kg} \cdot \text{m} \cdot \text{min}^{-1}}{6.12} = \dfrac{681 \text{ kg} \cdot \text{m} \cdot \text{min}^{-1}}{6.12} = \mathbf{111.27 \text{ W}}$

Stepping Equation

Stepping is used as both a mode of exercise testing and a form of rhythmic exercise. Step height is varied, but stepping typically involves a four-step process to complete a stepping cycle. One step is stepping forward and onto a box or bench, lifting the body and other leg onto the box, then stepping backward and down followed by the second leg. Oxygen cost is dependent on step rate and step height.

Derivation of the Stepping Equation

Similar to the walking and running up an incline equations, the stepping equation is composed of a horizontal component, a vertical component, and a resting component.

The horizontal component represents the cost of stepping forward and backward onto the box or bench. The oxygen cost of the complete cycle of stepping forward and back during the stepping cycle is ~0.2 mL · kg^{-1} body mass (0.2 mL · kg^{-1} · min^{-1}). Therefore, the horizontal component of stepping can be computed as:

$$\textbf{Horizontal component} = \text{Stepping rate (steps} \cdot \text{min}^{-1}) \times 0.2 \text{ mL} \cdot \text{kg}^{-1} \cdot \text{min}^{-1}$$

The vertical component represents the oxygen cost of both stepping up (1.8 mL · kg^{-1} · min^{-1}) and stepping down (1.33 mL · kg^{-1} · min^{-1}).

$$\textbf{Vertical component} = 1.33 \text{ mL} \cdot \text{kg}^{-1} \cdot \text{min}^{-1} \times [1.8 \text{ mL} \cdot \text{kg}^{-1} \cdot \text{min}^{-1} \times f \text{ (steps} \cdot \text{min}^{-1}) \times H \text{ (m)}]$$

$$\textbf{Resting component} = 3.5 \text{ mL} \cdot \text{kg}^{-1} \cdot \text{min}^{-1}$$

The ACSM's Stepping Equation

$$\dot{V}O_2 \text{ mL} \cdot \text{kg}^{-1} \cdot \text{min}^{-1} = [f \text{ (steps} \cdot \text{min}^{-1}) \times 0.2] + [1.33 \times 1.8 \times \text{Steps (steps} \cdot \text{min}^{-1}) \times H \text{ (m)}] + 3.5$$

- Note that f denotes stepping rate.
- Note that H denotes step height in meters.
  - When H is given in inches, the conversion factor is 1 in = 0.0254 m.

Limitations of the Stepping Equation

1. Steady-State Exercise Only!
   - The ACSM's stepping equation was computed based on steady-state oxygen consumption values. Therefore, the equation will not be as accurate when computing oxygen consumption during non–steady-state exercise.
2. Stepping rate and height
   - The accuracy of the stepping equation is highest between stepping rates of 12 and 30 steps · min^{-1} and step heights of 0.04 and 0.40 m (1.6–15.7 in).

Examples and Solutions for the Stepping Equation

1. Joe is stepping to a beat of 25 steps · min^{-1} on a step that is 7 in high. What is Joe's oxygen cost?
   - $\dot{V}O_2 \text{ mL} \cdot \text{kg}^{-1} \cdot \text{min}^{-1} = [f \text{ (steps} \cdot \text{min}^{-1}) \times 0.2] + [1.33 \times 1.8 \times \text{Steps (steps} \cdot \text{min}^{-1}) \times H \text{ (m)}] + 3.5$
     - Step height conversion: 7 in × 0.0254 = 0.178 m
   - $\dot{V}O_2 \text{ mL} \cdot \text{kg}^{-1} \cdot \text{min}^{-1} = [25 \times 0.2] + [1.33 \times 1.8 \times 25 \times 0.178] + 3.5$
   - $\dot{V}O_2 \text{ mL} \cdot \text{kg}^{-1} \cdot \text{min}^{-1} = 5 + 10.65 + 3.5 = \mathbf{19.15 \text{ mL} \cdot \text{kg}^{-1} \cdot \text{min}^{-1}}$

2. Alicia is prescribed an exercise intensity of 24.5 mL · kg^{-1} · min^{-1}. Using a 10-in step, calculate the desired step rate needed to equate to the prescribed intensity.
   - $\dot{V}O_2$ mL · kg^{-1} · min^{-1} = [f(steps · min^{-1}) × 0.2] + [1.33 × 1.8 × f(steps · min^{-1}) × H (m)] + 3.5
     - Step height conversion: 10 in × 0.0254 = 0.254 m
   - 24.5 mL · kg^{-1} · min^{-1} = [f × 0.2] + [1.33 × 1.8 × Steps × 0.254] + 3.5
     - Subtract 3.5 from both sides of the equation
   - 21 = [f × 0.2] + [1.33 × 1.8 × f × 0.254]
   - 21 = 0.2f + 0.61f = 0.81f
     - Divide both sides by 0.81
   - f = 25.93 = **26 steps · min^{-1}**

3. Richard is prescribed an exercise intensity of 20 mL · kg^{-1} · min^{-1}. Using a 30 steps · min^{-1} rate, calculate the step height needed to equate to the prescribed intensity.
   - $\dot{V}O_2$ mL · kg^{-1} · min^{-1} = [f(steps · min^{-1}) × 0.2] + [1.33 × 1.8 × f(steps · min^{-1}) × H (m)] + 3.5
   - 20 mL · kg^{-1} · min^{-1} = [30 × 0.2] + [1.33 × 1.8 × 30 × H] + 3.5
     - Subtract 3.5 from both sides of the equation
   - 16.5 = [f × 0.2] + [1.33 × 1.8 × 30 × H]
   - 16.5 = 6 + (71.82 × H)
     - Subtract 6 from both sides of the equation
   - 10.5 = 71.82H
     - Divide both sides by 71.82
   - H = 0.15 m
   - $H = \dfrac{0.15}{0.0254}$ = **5.9 in**

OTHER USEFUL EQUATIONS

In addition to the ACSM's metabolic equations, the exercise professional should also be aware of other equations that are being utilized to determine exercise intensity. These include HR$_{max}$, when a measurement is not available; the heart rate reserve (HRR); and oxygen uptake reserve ($\dot{V}O_2R$) methods (3).

Exercise Intensity Estimation Equations

Several methods for estimating exercise intensity are presented in Box 6.1. Intensity of aerobic exercise training is usually determined as a range, so the calculation using the formula presented in Box 6.1 needs to be repeated twice; one time for the lower limit of the desired intensity range and once for the upper limit of the desired intensity range. The prescribed exercise intensity range for an individual should be determined by taking various factors into consideration, including age, habitual PA level, physical fitness level, and health status (Table 6.2). The accuracy of any of these methods

Box 6.1	Summary of Methods for Prescribing Exercise Intensity Using Heart Rate (HR), Oxygen Uptake (O$_2$), and Metabolic Equivalents (METs)

- HRR method: Target HR = [(HR$_{max/peak}$ − HR$_{rest}$) × % intensity desired] + HR$_{rest}$
- $\dot{V}O_2R$ method: Target $\dot{V}O_2R$ = [($\dot{V}O_{2max/peak}$ − $\dot{V}O_{2rest}$) × % intensity desired + $\dot{V}O_{2rest}$
- HR method: Target HR = HR$_{max/peak}$ × % intensity desired
- $\dot{V}O_2$ method: Target $\dot{V}O_2$ = $\dot{V}O_{2max/peak}$ × % intensity desired
- MET method: Target MET = [($\dot{V}O_{2max/peak}$) / 3.5 mL · kg^{-1} · min^{-1}] × % intensity desired

HR$_{max/peak}$ is the highest value obtained during maximal/peak exercise or it can be estimated by 220 − age or some other prediction equation (7,8,9,10). $\dot{V}O_{2max/peak}$ is the highest value obtained during maximal/peak exercise or it can be estimated from a submaximal exercise test (3). Activities at the target $\dot{V}O_2$ and MET can be determined using a compendium of physical activity (11,12) or metabolic calculations (13). HR$_{max/peak}$, maximal or peak heart rate; HRR, heart rate reserve; HR$_{rest}$, resting heart rate; $\dot{V}O_{2max/peak}$, maximal or peak volume of oxygen consumed per unit of time; $\dot{V}O_2R$, oxygen uptake reserve; $\dot{V}O_{2rest}$, resting volume of oxygen consumed per unit of time.

TABLE 6.2 • Methods of Estimating Intensity of Cardiorespiratory Exercise

Relative Intensity

Intensity	%HRR or % $\dot{V}O_2R$	%HRmax	$\dot{V}O_2max$	Perceived Exertion (Rating on 6-20 RPE Scale)
Very light	<30	<57	<37	Very light (RPE < 9)
Light	30-39	57-63	37-45	Very light to fairly light (RPE 9-11)
Moderate	40-59	64-76	46-63	Fairly light to somewhat hard (RPE 12-13)
Vigorous	60-89	77-95	64-90	Somewhat hard to very hard (RPE 14-17)
Near-maximal to maximal	≥90	≥96	≥91	≥ Very hard (RPE ≥ 18)

HR_{max}, maximal heart rate; HRR, heart rate reserve; MET, metabolic equivalent; RPE, rating of perceived exertion; $\dot{V}O_{2max}$, maximum oxygen consumption; $\dot{V}O_2R$, oxygen uptake reserve.

Adapted from American College of Sports Medicine. *ACSM's Guidelines for Exercise Testing and Prescription.* 11th ed. Philadelphia (PA): Wolters Kluwer; 2021; Garber CE, Blissmer B, Deschenes MR, et al. Quantity and quality of exercise for developing and maintaining cardiorespiratory, musculoskeletal, and neuromotor fitness in apparently healthy adults: guidance for prescribing exercise. *Med Sci Sports Exerc.* 2011;43(7):1334-1359 (6).

may be influenced by the method of measurement or estimation used; therefore, direct measurement of the physiologic responses to exercise through an incremental (graded) cardiopulmonary exercise test is the preferred method for exercise prescription whenever possible (see Chapter 5). In addition, it is important to note that the HRR and the $\dot{V}O_2R$ methods are recommended for exercise prescription because exercise intensity can be underestimated or overestimated when using an HR-dependent method (*i.e.*, %HR_{max}) or $\dot{V}O_2$ (*i.e.*, %$\dot{V}O_{2max}$).

Examples and Solutions for Estimating Exercise Intensity

1. Jane's $\dot{V}O_{2max}$ from a graded exercise test was 21.5 mL $\cdot$ kg^{-1} $\cdot$ min^{-1}. Calculate an exercise intensity of 50% of her $\dot{V}O_{2max}$.
   - 21.5×0.50 (50%) = **10.75 mL $\cdot$ kg^{-1} $\cdot$ min^{-1}**
2. Jane's $\dot{V}O_{2max}$ from a graded exercise test was 21.5 mL $\cdot$ kg^{-1} $\cdot$ min^{-1}. Calculate an exercise intensity of 50% $\dot{V}O_2R$.
   - Target $\dot{V}O_2R = [(\dot{V}O_{2max/peak} - \dot{V}O_{2rest}) \times$ intensity desired] $+ \dot{V}O_{2rest}$
   - Target $\dot{V}O_2R = [21.5 - 3.5) \times 50\%] + 3.5$
   - Target $\dot{V}O_2R = [18 \times 0.50] + 3.5 = 9 + 3.5 =$ **12.5 mL $\cdot$ kg^{-1} $\cdot$ min^{-1}**

Jacob HR_{max} was measured during a graded exercise test and found to be 180 beats per min (bpm). Assuming Jacob's HR_{rest} is 70 ¯bpm, calculate his exercise intensity range, 50% to 60%, using the HRR method.

   - Target HR $= [(HR_{2max/peak} - HR_{2rest}) \times$ intensity desired] $+ HR_{2rest}$
   - Lower range
     - Target HR $= [(180 - 70) \times 50\%] + 70$
     - Target HR $= [110 \times 0.5] + 70 =$ **125 bpm**
   - Upper range
     - Target HR $= [(180 - 70) \times 60\%] + 70$
     - Target HR $= [110 \times 0.6] + 70 =$ **136 bpm**
   - Jacob's exercise intensity range is **125 to 136 bpm**.

SUMMARY

Energy requirements can be expressed in terms of the oxygen requirements of the PA being performed — commonly referred to as the oxygen consumption or oxygen cost ($\dot{V}O_2$). $\dot{V}O_2$ is perhaps best known as a maximal measure ($\dot{V}O_{2max}$) and provides useful information for exercise professionals of their participant's CRF. Exercise professionals may need to be able to calculate, by measuring or estimating, the energy requirements of various forms of PA to best advise their clients and to individualize the amount and type of PA needed to improve and maintain their participant's health.

PRACTICE PROBLEMS

The following 34 questions will require you to use all of the metabolic equations, as well as conversions to kilocalorie, METs, and other common transformations. The problems are grouped as mini-case studies, with three problems per case. You may need the results from one problem in order to accurately complete the next problem. All problems are worked to their correct solution at the end of the chapter.

A 75-kg man cycles at 120 W on the leg ergometer.

1. What is his training $\dot{V}O_2$?
   a. 24 METs
   b. 17.06 mL $\cdot$ kg^{-1} $\cdot$ min^{-1}
   c. 12.5 mL $\cdot$ kg^{-1} $\cdot$ min^{-1}
   d. 7 METs

2. What was his energy expenditure during a 30-minute ride?
   a. 277 kcal
   b. 9.2 kcal
   c. 1050 kcal
   d. 300 kcal

3. If he chooses to walk up a 10% grade, what is the appropriate walking speed?
   a. 211 m $\cdot$ min^{-1}
   b. 3.4 mph
   c. 2.8 mph
   d. 100 m $\cdot$ min^{-1}

During an aerobic dance class, Lisa, weighing 58 kg, is stepping on a 9-in step at a rate of 20 steps $\cdot$ min^{-}.

4. How many kilocalories will she expend in 20 minutes?
   a. 107
   b. 160
   c. 5.4
   d. 185

5. What is an equivalent work rate on the leg ergometer?
   a. 300 W
   b. 2264 W
   c. 120 kg $\cdot$ m $\cdot$ min^{-1}
   d. 370 kg $\cdot$ m $\cdot$ min^{-1}

An 80-kg male is running on a level track at 9 mph.

6. What is his $\dot{V}O_2$?
   a. 51.7 mL $\cdot$ kg^{-1} $\cdot$ min^{-1}
   b. 10 METs
   c. 27.6 mL $\cdot$ kg^{-1} $\cdot$ min^{-1}
   d. 42.3 mL $\cdot$ kg^{-1} $\cdot$ min^{-1}

7. How many calories per minute is he expending?
   a. 0.11 kcal $\cdot$ min^{-1}
   b. 50 kcal $\cdot$ min^{-1}
   c. 20.5 kcal $\cdot$ min^{-1}
   d. 7.5 kcal $\cdot$ min^{-1}

John's $\dot{V}O_2$max is 32 mL $\cdot$ kg^{-1} $\cdot$ min^{-1}. He weighs 74 kg.

8. What is his work rate on the Monark arm ergometer at 40% of $\dot{V}O_{2ax}$?
   a. 703 kg $\cdot$ m $\cdot$ min^{-1}
   b. 688 kg $\cdot$ m $\cdot$ min^{-1}
   c. 100 kg $\cdot$ m $\cdot$ min^{-1}
   d. 229 kg $\cdot$ m $\cdot$ min^{-1}

9. What is his work rate on a leg ergometer at 80% of $\dot{V}O_2R$?
   a. 764 kg · m · min^{-1}
   b. 793 kg · m · min^{-1}
   c. 195 W
   d. 110 W

10. How many calories are expended at an exercise intensity of 60% of $\dot{V}O_{2max}$?
    a. 7.1 kcal · min^{-1}
    b. 11.8 kcal · min^{-1}
    c. 7.6 kcal · min^{-1}
    d. 9.2 kcal · min^{-1}

Nickole, a 54-kg woman, wants to begin a cross training program.

11. What is her $\dot{V}O_2$ at 2.5 mph and 12%?
    a. 1525 L · min^{-1}
    b. 6 METs
    c. 12 METs
    d. 24.7 mL · kg^{-1} · min^{-1}

12. What is the equivalent work rate on the cycle ergometer?
    a. 30 W
    b. 531 kg · m · min^{-1}
    c. 575 kg · m · min^{-1}
    d. 87 kg · m · min^{-1}

13. If she steps on a 12-in step, what step rate is required to elicit the same $\dot{V}O_2$?
    a. 23 steps · min^{-1}
    b. 20 steps · min^{-1}
    c. 27 steps · min^{-1}
    d. 30 steps · min^{-1}

On the Monark leg ergometer (flywheel 6 m · rev^{-1}), Dawn is cycling at 65 rev · min^{-1} against a load of 2 kg. She weighs 55 kg.

14. What is her $\dot{V}O_2$?
    a. 27 mL · kg^{-1} · min^{-1}
    b. 36 METs
    c. 1.8 L · min^{-1}
    d. 920 mL · min^{-1}

15. With an estimated $\dot{V}O_{2ax}$ of 3 L · min^{-1}, you determine a training intensity of 70% of $\dot{V}O_2R$ for Dawn. What is her corresponding work rate?
    a. 2.1 kg
    b. 161 W
    c. 143 W
    d. 1452 kg · m · min^{-1}

16. Dawn's preferred intensity for jogging is 6.5 mph. What is her corresponding $\dot{V}O_2$ at this intensity?
    a. 34.6 mL · kg^{-1} · min^{-1}
    b. 11 METs
    c. 6.5 METs
    d. 2.5 L · min^{-1}

Steve is working out on the Monark arm ergometer (flywheel 2.4 m · rev^{-1}). The resistance is set at 1.5 kg, and he is cranking at 60 rev · min^{-1}. He weighs 85 kg.

17. What is his estimated energy expenditure?
    a. 4.7 kcal · min^{-1}
    b. 9.6 kcal · min^{-1}
    c. 7.4 kcal · min^{-1}
    d. 8 kcal · min^{-1}

18. Moving to stepping, Steve steps on a 10-in box at 24 steps · min^{-1}. What is his estimated energy expenditure?
    a. 9.6 kcal · min^{-1}
    b. 4.7 kcal · min^{-1}
    c. 11.3 kcal · min^{-1}
    d. 6.1 kcal · min^{-1}

19. Completing his circuit, Steve walks on the treadmill at 3.5 mph up a 12% incline. What is his estimated energy expenditure?
    a. 11.3 kcal · min^{-1}
    b. 13.2 kcal · min^{-1}
    c. 14.1 kcal · min^{-1}
    d. 9.6 kcal · min^{-1}

Otto, a client in your cardiac rehab program, needs a circuit exercise intensity prescription. His functional capacity is 8 METs. He weighs 90 kg.

20. What is his arm ergometer work rate at 40% of his MET capacity?
    a. 11.2 W
    b. 73.5 kg · m · min^{-1}
    c. 75 kg · m · min^{-1}
    d. 231 kg · m · min^{-1}

21. Cycling (leg) at 65% of $\dot{V}O_2R$, how many kilocalories is he expending?
    a. 8.7 kcal · min^{-1}
    b. 5.5 kcal · min^{-1}
    c. 19.4 kcal · min^{-1}
    d. 14.2 kcal · min^{-1}

22. Walking at 50% of $\dot{V}O_{2ax}$, his speed is 3 mph. What is the required grade?
    a. 2.5%
    b. 1.7%
    c. 3%
    d. 2%

Your client, Jim, is interested in weight control. He weighs 75 kg.

23. If Jim walks 3.3 mph, how long must he walk to expend the 300 kcal?
    a. 52 minutes
    b. 42 minutes
    c. 65 minutes
    d. 99 minutes

24. If Jim exercises at an intensity equivalent to 6 kcal · min^{-1}, what is the leg ergometer work rate?
    a. 47 W
    b. 90 W
    c. 61 W
    d. 71 W

25. Cycling on the arm ergometer at 1 kg and 50 rev · min^{-1}, how long would it take Jim to expend 300 kcal (assume 2.4 m per pedal rev)?
    a. 1 hour 37 minutes
    b. 52 minutes
    c. 1 hour
    d. 1 hour 14 minutes

An exercise test was performed on a triathlete. His $\dot{V}O_2max$ was 73 mL · kg^{-1} · min^{-1}. He weighs 73 kg.

26. His anaerobic threshold was 80% of $\dot{V}O_{2max}$. What is his running speed at his threshold?
    a. 10 min · mi^{-1} pace
    b. 58.4 m · s^{-1}
    c. 10.2 mph
    d. 200 m · min^{-1}

27. His leg ergometer work rate is typically 1100 kg · m · min^{-1}. What percent of $\dot{V}O_{2max}$ is this?
    a. 39%
    b. 47%
    c. 34%
    d. 60%

28. To train for hills, you have him run at a $\dot{V}O_2$ of 50 mL · kg^{-1} · min^{-1} up a 5% incline. What is the appropriate running speed?
    a. 190 m · min^{-1}
    b. 9 min · mi^{-1} pace
    c. 90 m · s^{-1}
    d. 9 mph

You allow your client, Lisa, to self-select training intensity. She weighs 55 kg.

29. If she cycles on the Monark leg ergometer against a 1.5 kg resistance at 75 rev · min^{-1}, what is her $\dot{V}O_2$?
    a. 22.1 mL · kg^{-1} · min^{-1}
    b. 12 METs
    c. 9.8 mL · kg^{-1} · min^{-1}
    d. 8.3 METs

30. She wants to replicate the same intensity as the previous question, but by walking on the treadmill up a 10% incline. What is the appropriate walking speed?
    a. 2.5 mph
    b. 4 mph
    c. 1.7 mph
    d. 3.4 mph

31. How many kilocalories will she expend during a 30-minute workout?
    a. 240
    b. 80
    c. 8
    d. 15

Your client completes the Bruce treadmill protocol and has an estimated $\dot{V}O_2$max of 12 METs. She weighs 47 kg.

32. If she cranks the arm ergometer against a 2 kg resistance at 50 rev · min^{-1}, at what percent of $\dot{V}O_{2max}$ is she working?
    a. 50%
    b. 45%
    c. 55%
    d. 60%

33. If you want her to work at 50% of her $\dot{V}O_2R$ by stepping on a 15-in step, what is her step rate?
    a. 15 steps · min^{-1}
    b. 17 steps · min^{-1}
    c. 20 steps · min^{-1}
    d. 12 steps · min^{-1}

34. Working at 7 METs, how many minutes must she exercise in order to expend 200 kcal?
    a. 35
    b. 60
    c. 20
    d. 42

ANSWERS

1 d	8 d	15 b	22 b	29 d
2 a	9 b	16 b	23 c	30 d
3 c	10 a	17 a	24 c	31 a
4 a	11 d	18 a	25 a	32 b
5 d	12 b	19 c	26 c	33 b
6 a	13 a	20 d	27 b	34 a
7 c	14 c	21 a	28 a	

REFERENCES

1. U.S. Department of Health and Human Services. *Physical Activity Guidelines for Americans*. 2nd ed. 2018 [cited 2020 Jan 21]. Available from: https://health.gov/paguidelines/second-edition/pdf/Physical_Activity_Guidelines_2nd_edition.pdf.
2. Kenney WL, Wilmore JH, Costill DL. *Physiology of Sport and Exercise*. 7th ed. Champaign: Human Kinetics; 2019.
3. American College of Sports Medicine. *ACSM's Guidelines for Exercise Testing and Prescription*. 11th ed. Philadelphia (PA): Wolters Kluwer; 2021.
4. Swain DP, Brawner CA. *Medicine ACoS. ACSM's Resource Manual for Guidelines for Exercise Testing and Prescription*. 7th ed. Philadelphia (PA): Wolters Kluwer Health/Lippincott Williams & Wilkins; 2014.
5. Whaley MH, Brubaker PH, Otto RM, Armstrong LE. *ACSM's Guidelines for Exercise Testing and Prescription*. 7th ed. Philadelphia (PA): Lippincott Williams & Wilkins; 2006.
6. Garber CE, Blissmer B, Deschenes MR, et al. Quantity and quality of exercise for developing and maintaining cardiorespiratory, musculoskeletal, and neuromotor fitness in apparently healthy adults: guidance for prescribing exercise. *Med Sci Sports Exerc*. 2011;43(7):1334–59.
7. Åstrand, Irma, Per-Olof Åstrand, and Kaare Rodahl. "Maximal heart rate during work in older men. *J Appl Physiol*. 1959; 14(4):562–6.
8. Tanaka H, Monahan KD, Seals DR. Age-predicted maximal heart rate revisited. *J Am Coll Cardiol*. 2001;37(1):153–6.
9. Gellish RL, Goslin BR, Olson RE, McDonald A, Russi GD, Moudgil VK. Longitudinal modeling of the relationship between age and maximal heart rate. *Med Sci Sports Exerc*. 2007;39(5):822–9.
10. Gulati M, Shaw LJ, Thisted RA, Black HR, Merz CNB, Arnsdorf MF. Heart rate response to exercise stress testing in asymptomatic women: the st. James women take heart project. *Circulation*. 2010;122(2): 130–37
11. Ainsworth BE, Haskell WL, Leon AS, et al. Compendium of physical activities: classification of energy costs of human physical activities. *Med Sci Sports Exerc*. 1993;25(1):71–80.
12. Ainsworth BE, Haskell WL, Whitt MC, et al. Compendium of physical activities: an update of activity codes and MET intensities. *Med Sci Sports Exerc*. 2000;32(9):S498–516.
13. Glass S, Dwyer GB. *ACSM'S Metabolic Calculations Handbook*. Philadelphia (PA): Lippincott Williams & Wilkins; 2007.

CHAPTER 7

Muscular Fitness

WHY MEASURE MUSCULAR FITNESS

Muscular fitness is well accepted as a critical component of good physical function. The ACSM combines the functional parameters of strength, endurance, and power to described muscular fitness (1). Most routine daily tasks require some aspect of muscular fitness, whether lifting a household object, performing yard work, or participating in a recreational sport. Further, as participants age, muscular fitness becomes even more important for many reasons, including the ability to continue living independently and to avoid the deleterious effects of sarcopenia, which further reduces functional ability and quality of life. In addition, improved muscular fitness results in improved posture, decreased risk of musculoskeletal injuries, better bone mass (decreased risk of osteoporosis), improved glucose uptake (better blood glucose control), and potentially increased resting metabolic rate (better body weight control).

In order to evaluate a participant's overall muscular fitness, a comprehensive muscular fitness assessment should be carried out. This type of muscular fitness evaluation allows an exercise professional to establish a baseline measure for participant, which can then serve as a benchmark of future progress. The *2018 Physical Activity Guidelines for Americans* recommends that both children and adults complete "muscle-strengthening activities of moderate or greater intensity on multiple days of the week" (2). Therefore, when following these guidelines, it would be prudent to begin with an assessment of muscular fitness, regardless of whether working with children, older adults, or participants with chronic disease (with appropriate modifications as designated by one's health care provider).

UNIQUE ASSESSMENT PRINCIPLES

Muscular strength, endurance, and power are measurable components of physical fitness. Overall, *muscular strength* refers to the muscle's ability to exert a maximal force on one occasion, *muscular endurance* is the muscle's ability to continue to perform successive exertions or repetitions against a submaximal load, and *muscular power* is the muscle's ability to exert force per unit of time (*i.e.*, rate) (3). One unique aspect of muscle measurement is that there are approximately 700 skeletal muscles in the human body, each of which can yield a different level of performance. So, unlike body composition and cardiorespiratory endurance, there is no one universal measure that provides an assessment of a individual's muscular fitness. Then, to further complicate the assessment of muscular fitness, there are two distinct types of muscular contractions, each requiring unique types of assessments. In addition, most muscular contractions involve more than one muscle; therefore, performance can vary with technique and variation of the method employed to load the muscle. Because myriad factors can influence muscular strength and muscular endurance, finding any one assessment is not possible (4).

Another consideration when performing assessments of muscular fitness is the differences that one will encounter among individuals, particularly, differences in their body weight, skill level, fitness level, and even their respective motivation to perform any particular assessment.

Types of Contractions

There are two principal types of muscular contractions: static and dynamic. During a static contraction, the muscle generates force (*i.e.*, contraction) without movement taking place. This may involve pushing or pulling against an immovable object or holding an object in place. This type of contraction is also called *isometric* ("iso" meaning equal and "metric" meaning length) because the length of the muscle does not change during the execution of the contraction.

Dynamic contractions are those that generate force with an associated change in muscle length. The muscle length changes are either eccentric, when the muscle lengthens, or concentric, when the muscle shortens. In addition, if the movement involves a fixed amount of resistance, it is called an *isotonic contraction*; and if movement takes place at a fixed speed, it is termed an *isokinetic contraction*. The reader is encouraged to further review these terms in any of the several exercise physiology text currently available.

Familiarization

Some assessment procedures for muscular fitness may require tasks that are uncommon and infrequently performed by the participant and therefore require a familiarization period. Like many other activities, performance can be improved through becoming familiar with the activity and practicing a technique; this familiarization process is known as a *learning effect*. Thus, for a muscular fitness assessment to accurately reflect the ability of any given participant, a reasonable period of time to allow for the learning effect to take place is necessary. Failure to allow for this familiarization will negatively impact the assessment results.

Participant performance is also related to the opportunity for a warm-up period before participation in the muscular fitness assessments. In all, 5 to 10 minutes of light-intensity aerobic exercise (*e.g.*, treadmill or cycle) is recommended, followed by several low-intensity repetitions of the exercise being tested. Beyond the physiologic factors of increasing blood circulation to the muscles and increasing the temperature of the muscles, a warm-up allows a neurologic familiarization refresher immediately before the assessment. It is worth noting, however, that the familiarization and the warm-up period should be different times, because they have different purposes for the participant.

Method of Loading

Free weights and resistance exercise machines are the two major sources of resistance to the muscle for dynamic contractions. Each has advantages and disadvantages, both for assessment and training. Some of the advantages for free weights are uniformity (*i.e.*, a 25-lb weight plate is the same at every facility), the wide range of movement patterns that can be performed, and the similarity of movement to everyday activities (*e.g.*, lifting and putting a weighted object on an overhead shelf). The disadvantages to free weights for assessment purposes are potential difficulty in isolating a muscle group, safety issues related to possibly dropping the weights, and coordination issues, which may lead to injury.

Resistance exercise machines with supported weights, as shown in Figure 7.1, provide some advantages over free weights. One advantage is the ability to better isolate a muscle group, which allows for a more precise muscular assessment. Another advantage is the minimized risk associated with the possibility of being injured from dropping a weight. However, disadvantages of resistance exercise machines should be considered because they limit movement patterns to one per machine. This limitation may be important to consider when testing participants with limited range of motion.

The isolated movement patterns are not necessarily typical of everyday activities, and significant variability can exist in the designated amount of weight between different brands of machines (*e.g.*, some machines only use a 1, 2, 3, 4 . . . system to designate a difference in load vs. actual pounds lifted). In addition, many machines have some type of mechanism that varies the resistance applied throughout the range of motion of the contraction, with different manufacturers' having different mechanisms to vary the resistance (cams, levers, pulleys, etc.). Obviously, these differences create difficulties in comparing results from assessments performed on different resistance exercise machines, which is not an issue with free weights. The ability to track the participant over the course of many years can also be affected if the machines used by a facility are upgraded with new models or if a participant joins a new facility with different machines.

In muscular endurance testing, some of the assessments use the participant's body weight as the source of the resistance. In addition, some tests employ a fixed amount of absolute weight, whereas

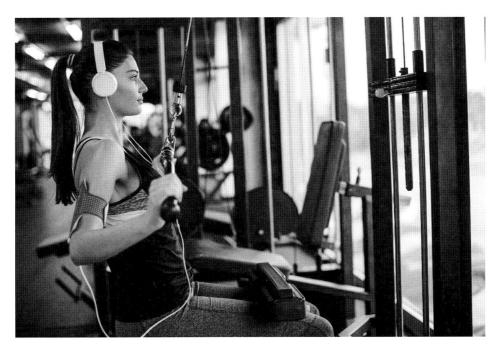

Figure 7.1 An example of a resistance exercise unit that uses a weight stack for loading.

others may use a fixed percentage of a person's maximum capacity. Depending on the method used to select the resistance, the outcome will vary.

Proper Positioning

Proper positioning is essential for assessments using either free weights or machines. Standardization of the positioning allows for accurate measurement of the muscle group being assessed and for reliable retesting over time. Variations in positioning can potentially allow other muscle groups to contribute to movement of the load, which will likely increase the amount of weight recorded for the assessment, thereby producing inaccurate results. In addition, proper positioning may be necessary for the safety of the participant.

Specificity

The principle of specificity is most typically applied to exercise training where an exercise program has been tailored to precisely mimic a specific performance goal or activity. Specificity also has relevance for assessment because each muscle group tested will have different capabilities depending on the specific requirements of the test methodology. The strength or endurance of a muscle will be specific to the size of the muscle and limb, the type of contraction, the exact movement pattern (or the joint angle for a static measure), the speed of the movement, and the amount of resistance. Because these specificity characteristics vary among different muscular fitness assessment procedures, interpretation of test results becomes challenging. One key for an assessment of muscular fitness is standardization within the measurement procedure.

MUSCULAR FITNESS CONTINUUM

Muscular fitness exists along a continuum with muscular strength and muscular endurance at opposite ends (Figure 7.2). From an assessment perspective, strength is the measurement of the maximal force capability of the muscle, and endurance is the measurement of the ability to continue performing contractions at a submaximal level. As the needs of a given task move closer to the center of the continuum, the contribution of both muscle endurance and muscle strength become more equal. Even though muscular power may not fit within this continuum, it is an important parameter to evaluate because muscular power declines at a faster rate than muscular strength or muscular endurance with aging (5), and it may be the most valuable muscular fitness variables for predicting maintenance of functional independence and improving quality of life (6).

STRENGTH ASSESSMENTS

It is important to note that before beginning any assessment, it is important the participant has provided consent and, at a minimum, a Physical Activity Readiness Questionnaire for Everyone (PAR-Q+) has been provided as a screening tool. The assessment of muscular strength will be specific to the muscle group and the other unique assessment factors reviewed earlier. Thus, there is no one single measure of muscular strength for a participant. The suggested approach for the assessment of muscular strength is to use a variety of assessments of different muscles to capture a concept of a participant's overall muscle strength. However, attempting to create a "composite score" of strength would be limited in the case of a person with excellent strength levels in some muscles and poor strength levels in other muscles because this would lead to an inaccurate interpretation of "average" overall muscle strength.

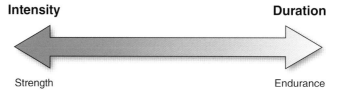

Figure 7.2 Strength-endurance continuum.

One important decision to be made in regard to measuring muscle strength involves selecting the best method of resistance for the assessments. This decision will be dictated, in part, by the interpretation scale to be used (*i.e.*, if the norms were developed from free weights, then free weights should be used for the assessment) and, of course, the availability of different types of assessment equipment.

Static

Static measures have long been used to assess muscle strength, with handgrip strength the most widely used. Static measures of muscular strength use either dynamometers or tensiometers, which are durable types of equipment that come at a relatively low cost, thereby making these tests popular.

Dynamometers

The most commonly performed static strength test is the measurement of grip strength using a handgrip dynamometer. Even though the grip strength test is considered a "common test," its implications are important, as changes in grip strength provide evidence of skeletal muscle changes that occur over time (7,8), and reduced handgrip strength has been linked with diabetes, frailty, premature mortality (9), and even cognitive decline (10). Grip strength norms are given in Table 7.1, and the procedures for the grip strength test are described in Box 7.1 and illustrated in Figure 7.3.

TABLE 7.1 • Fitness Categories for Grip Strength[a] by Sex and Age

Age	5th	10th	25th	50th	75th	90th	95th
Males							
20-24	32	34	38	43	48	52	55
25-29	34	37	41	45	50	54	57
30-34	36	38	42	47	52	56	59
35-39	37	39	43	48	53	57	60
40-44	37	40	44	48	53	57	60
45-49	37	39	43	48	53	57	60
50-54	36	39	43	47	52	56	59
55-59	34	37	41	46	50	54	57
60-64	32	35	39	44	48	52	55
65-69	29	32	36	41	45	49	52
70-74	25	29	33	38	42	46	49
75-79	21	25	29	34	38	42	44
Females							
20-24	20	22	24	27	29	32	34
25-29	21	22	25	28	30	33	35
30-34	22	23	25	28	31	34	35
35-39	22	23	26	28	31	34	36
40-44	22	23	26	29	31	34	36
45-49	22	23	25	28	31	34	36
50-54	21	23	25	28	31	33	35
55-59	20	22	24	27	30	32	34
60-64	19	21	23	26	29	31	33
65-69	17	19	22	25	27	30	31
70-74	15	18	21	23	25	28	29
75-79	13	16	19	21	23	26	27

[a]Norms use the best score in kg for the left or right hands.

Box 7.1	Procedures for the Static Handgrip Strength Test

1. Have the participant stand for the test. Usually, this test is performed with each hand. The norms provided use a combined score for the right and left hands. The test can also be performed with only the dominant hand.
2. Adjust the grip bar so that the second joint of the fingers will be bent to grip the handle of the dynamometer.
3. Have the participant hold the handgrip dynamometer perpendicular to the side of the body. The elbow should be extended. Make sure that the dynamometer is set to zero.
4. The participant should then squeeze the handgrip dynamometer as hard as possible without holding the breath (to avoid the Valsalva maneuver). It is optional if the participant wishes to extend the elbow; however, other body movement should be avoided.
5. Record the grip strength in kilograms. Repeat this procedure using the opposite hand.
6. Repeat the test two more times with each hand. Take the highest of the three readings for each hand and add these two values (one from each hand) together as the measure of handgrip strength to compare with the norms presented in Table 7.1.

Another dynamometer test used in fitness settings is the assessment of static back and leg strength. An example of the type of dynamometer used for this assessment is shown in Figure 7.4.

Tensiometers

One form of static strength assessment employs a cable tensiometer that can be used to test multiple joint angles through a range of motion for a particular muscular contraction. Tensiometers can be mounted to walls or tables and set up to mimic various common activities. Tensiometers are more popular in sports-related physical fitness and therefore are not discussed in more detail in this chapter.

Dynamic

As reviewed earlier, dynamic muscular contractions are those in which the length of the muscle changes and can be performed with either concentric or eccentric movements and with different methods of loading the resistance.

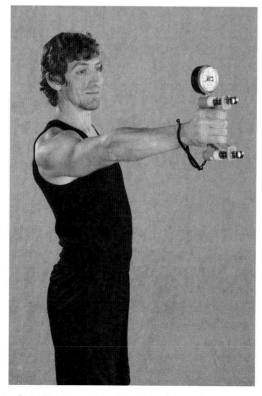

Figure 7.3 Measurement of static strength with a handgrip dynamometer.

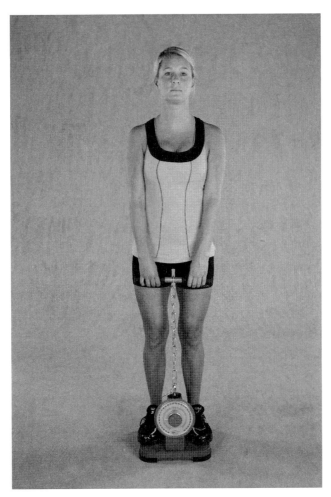

Figure 7.4 Measurement of back strength with a dynamometer.

Repetition Maximum

Repetition maximum (RM) is a term used to describe the maximal amount of weight that can be lifted through a full range of motion with good form. The one RM (1-RM) is typically considered the gold-standard measure of muscular strength (12). Although strength assessment protocols using multiple repetitions (*e.g.*, 4-RM, 6-RM, 8-RM) do exist (13,14), and there are some equations to predict a 1-RM value from these multiple RM tests (15), there are no clear standards or norms available for these evaluations.

The 1-RM test can be performed with any muscle group and can be tested using either free weights or machines. The procedures for performing a 1-RM assessment are provided in Box 7.2. The bench press, as a general measure of upper body strength, and the leg press, as a measure for lower body strength, are the two most common dynamic assessments used today. Tables 7.2 and 7.3 provide normative reference data for these two tests.

Box 7.2	**Procedures for a One Repetition Maximum (1-RM) Assessment (13,16,17)**

1. The participant should warm up by completing several submaximal repetitions.
2. Determine the 1-RM (or any multiple RM) within four trials with rest periods of 3 to 5 minutes between trials.
3. Select an initial weight that is within the subject's perceived capacity (~50%–70% of capacity).
4. Progressively increase resistance by 2.5 to 20 kg until the participant cannot complete the selected repetition(s); all repetitions should be performed at the same speed of movement and range of motion to ensure consistency between trials.
5. Record the final weight lifted successfully as the absolute 1-RM or multiple RM.

From Gibson AL, Wagner DR, Heyward VH. *Principles of Assessment, Prescription, and Exercise Program Adherence. Advanced Fitness Assessment and Exercise Prescription.* 8th ed. Champaign (IL): Human Kinetics; 2019. p. 56.

TABLE 7.2 • Fitness Categories for Upper Body Strength[a] for Men and Women by Age

Bench press weight ratio = weight pushed in lb/body weight in lb

Men

Percentile		<20	20-29	30-39	40-49	50-59	60+
				Age (yr)			
99	Superior	>1.76	>1.63	>1.35	>1.20	>1.05	>0.94
95	Superior	1.76	1.63	1.35	1.20	1.05	0.94
90		1.46	1.48	1.24	1.10	0.97	0.89
85	Excellent	1.38	1.37	1.17	1.04	0.93	0.84
80		1.34	1.32	1.12	1.00	0.90	0.82
75		1.29	1.26	1.08	0.96	0.87	0.79
70		1.24	1.22	1.04	0.93	0.84	0.77
65	Good	1.23	1.18	1.01	0.90	0.81	0.74
60		1.19	1.14	0.98	0.88	0.79	0.72
55		1.16	1.10	0.96	0.86	0.77	0.70
50		1.13	1.06	0.93	0.84	0.75	0.68
45	Fair	1.10	1.03	0.90	0.82	0.73	0.67
40		1.06	0.99	0.88	0.80	0.71	0.66
35		1.01	0.96	0.86	0.78	0.70	0.65
30	Poor	0.96	0.93	0.83	0.76	0.68	0.63
25		0.93	0.90	0.81	0.74	0.66	0.60
20		0.89	0.88	0.78	0.72	0.63	0.57
15		0.86	0.84	0.75	0.69	0.60	0.56
10	Very poor	0.81	0.80	0.71	0.65	0.57	0.53
5		0.76	0.72	0.65	0.59	0.53	0.49
1		<0.76	<0.72	<0.65	<0.59	<0.53	<0.49
N		60	425	1909	2090	1279	343

Total n = 6106

Bench press weight ratio = weight pushed in lb/body weight in lb

Women

Percentile		<20	20-29	30-39	40-49	50-59	60+
				Age (yr)			
99	Superior	>0.88	>1.01	>0.82	>0.77	>0.68	>0.72
95	Superior	0.88	1.01	0.82	0.77	0.68	0.72
90		0.83	0.90	0.76	0.71	0.61	0.64
85	Excellent	0.81	0.83	0.72	0.66	0.57	0.59
80		0.77	0.80	0.70	0.62	0.55	0.54
75		0.76	0.77	0.65	0.60	0.53	0.53
70		0.74	0.74	0.63	0.57	0.52	0.51
65	Good	0.70	0.72	0.62	0.55	0.50	0.48
60		0.65	0.70	0.60	0.54	0.48	0.47
55		0.64	0.68	0.58	0.53	0.47	0.46
50		0.63	0.65	0.57	0.52	0.46	0.45
45	Fair	0.60	0.63	0.55	0.51	0.45	0.44
40		0.58	0.59	0.53	0.50	0.44	0.43
35		0.57	0.58	0.52	0.48	0.43	0.41
30	Poor	0.56	0.56	0.51	0.47	0.42	0.40
25		0.55	0.53	0.49	0.45	0.41	0.39
20		0.53	0.51	0.47	0.43	0.39	0.38
15		0.52	0.50	0.45	0.42	0.38	0.36
10	Very poor	0.50	0.48	0.42	0.38	0.37	0.33
5		0.41	0.44	0.39	0.35	0.31	0.26
1		<0.41	<0.44	<0.39	<0.35	<0.31	<0.26
N		20	191	379	333	189	42

Total n = 1154

[a]One repetition maximum (1-RM) bench press, with bench press weight ratio = weight pushed in pounds/ body weight in pounds. 1-RM was measured using a universal dynamic variable resistance (DVR) machine.

Adapted with permission from Physical Fitness Assessments and Norms for Adults and Law Enforcement. Dallas, TX: The Cooper Institute; 2009. For more information: www.cooperinstitute.org.

TABLE 7.3 • Fitness Categories for Leg Strength by Age and Sex[a]

Leg press weight ratio = weight pushed in lb/body weight in lb

Percentile		Age (yr)				
		20–29	30–39	40–49	50–59	60+
Men						
90	Well above average	2.27	2.07	1.92	1.80	1.73
80	Above average	2.13	1.93	1.82	1.71	1.62
70		2.05	1.85	1.74	1.64	1.56
60	Average	1.97	1.77	1.68	1.58	1.49
50		1.91	1.71	1.62	1.52	1.43
40	Below average	1.83	1.65	1.57	1.46	1.38
30		1.74	1.59	1.51	1.39	1.30
20	Well below average	1.63	1.52	1.44	1.32	1.25
10		1.51	1.43	1.35	1.22	1.16
Women						
90	Well above average	1.82	1.61	1.48	1.37	1.32
80	Above average	1.68	1.47	1.37	1.25	1.18
70		1.58	1.39	1.29	1.17	1.13
60	Average	1.50	1.33	1.23	1.10	1.04
50		1.44	1.27	1.18	1.05	0.99
40	Below average	1.37	1.21	1.13	0.99	0.93
30		1.27	1.15	1.08	0.95	0.88
20	Well below average	1.22	1.09	1.02	0.88	0.85
10		1.14	1.00	0.94	0.78	0.72

[a]One repetition maximum (1-RM) leg press with leg press weight ratio = weight pushed/body weight.

Study population for the data set was predominantly white and college educated. A Universal Dynamic Variable Resistance (DVR) machine was used to measure the 1-repetition maximum (RM).

Adapted from Institute for Aerobics Research, Dallas, 1994.

Isokinetic

Isokinetic (contraction at a constant velocity) assessments of muscular fitness require specialized and expensive equipment. These assessments can include a wide range of data (*e.g.*, maximal tension throughout a complete range of motion) that prove highly reliable and accurate. These tests are commonly performed in both athletic and physical therapy rehabilitative programs. However, because of the cost of the equipment and the relatively long time period required to complete an assessment of one muscle group, this type of assessment is not commonly performed in a commercial fitness facility.

ENDURANCE ASSESSMENTS

Like muscular strength assessment, the assessment of muscular endurance will be specific to the muscle group and the other unique assessment factors reviewed earlier. Endurance assessments can be conducted by performing a fixed amount of contractions in a defined time period, performing a maximal number of contractions of a set resistance, or by holding a static contraction for a period of time. If the total number of repetitions at a given amount of resistance is measured, the result is termed *absolute muscular endurance*. If the number of repetitions performed at a percentage of the 1-RM (*e.g.*, 70%) is used pre-testing and post-testing, the result is termed *relative muscular endurance*.

1. The participant stands on a movable box positioned beneath the bar and grasps the bar with an overhand grip (palms facing away) in a position in which the chin is above the bar, elbows are flexed, and the chest is next to the bar.
2. With the participant grasping the bar, the box is slid away and a stopwatch is started.
3. The position is held as long as possible.
4. The time is stopped when the chin touches the bar and dips below the bar or the head tilts back to keep the chin above the bar.

Static

One option for muscular endurance assessment is the use of timed tests of holding a submaximal contraction. One long-used static test for muscular endurance is the timed flexed arm hang. The procedure for this test is provided in Box 7.3; standards for youth and military personnel exist (President's Challenge and U.S. Marine Corps.); however, true national norms for adults are lacking.

A static endurance test used for core strength is the prone plank hold (see Figure 7.5). Percentile rank scores do exist for the plank test; however, true national norms for adults are still lacking. Procedures for the plank test are provided in Box 7.4.

Dynamic

Dynamic tests of muscular endurance can be performed with free weights, resistance exercise machines, or using callisthenic-type exercises. This section covers some of the more common endurance tests for which normative values exist. However, fitness professionals often create their own tests that can be used as serial assessments over time with a participant, assuming they are easily repeatable.

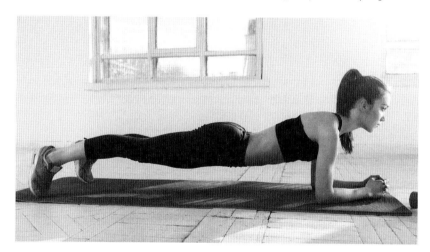

Figure 7.5 Prone plank hold.

Box 7.4	Procedures for the Prone Plank Test

1. Participant assumes the forearm plank position with elbows in contact with the ground such that the humerus forms a perpendicular line to the horizontal plane, directly beneath the shoulders.
2. The forearms are in the neutral position with hands directly in front of the elbows.
3. The participant assumes a rigid anatomical body position so that only their forearms and toes support the body.
4. This position is characterized by a phalangeal extension, neutral ankle position, knee and hip extension, and neutral spinal positions.
5. The participant holds this position as long as possible.
6. The test is terminated when (a) the participant voluntarily stops the test, (b) the participant failed to maintain the proper position, (c) the participant reports ill effects from the test (*e.g.*, headache, dizziness, pain not associated with fatigue), or (d) the test ends.

From US Department of Health and Human Services. *Physical Activity Guidelines for Americans*. Washington (DC): Department of Health and Human Services; 2018. Available from: https://health.gov/paguidelines/second-edition/.

Box 7.5   Push-Up Test Procedures for Measurement of Muscular Endurance

Push-Up

1. The push-up test is administered with male subjects starting in the standard "down" position (hands pointing forward and under the shoulder, back straight, head up, using the toes as the pivotal point) and female subjects in the modified "knee push-up" position (legs together, lower leg in contact with mat with ankles plantar flexed, back straight, hands shoulder width apart, head up, using the knees as the pivotal point).
2. The participant must raise the body by straightening the elbows and return to the "down" position, until the chin touches the mat. The stomach should not touch the mat.
3. For both men and women, the participant's back must be straight at all times, and the participant must push up to a straight arm position.
4. The maximal number of push-ups performed consecutively without rest is counted as the score.
5. The test is stopped when the participant strains forcibly or is unable to maintain the appropriate technique within two repetitions.

Results are compared with the norms presented in Table 7.4.

Push-Up Test

The push-up test can be used to assess muscular endurance in men and women alike. There are sex-specific protocols for the push-up (Box 7.5; Figure 7.6), and regardless of protocol, the maximum

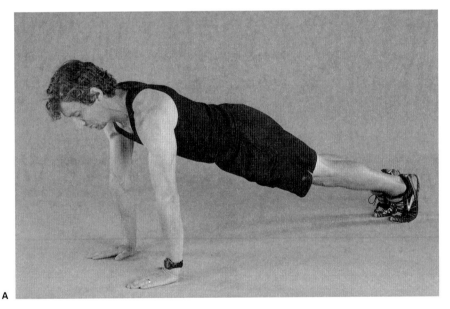

A

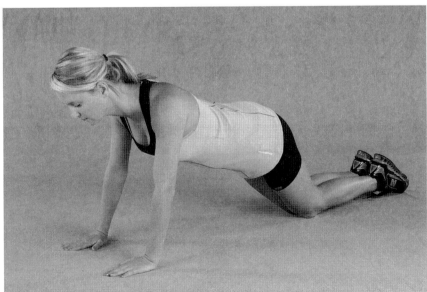

B

Figure 7.6 Different starting positions for men (**A**) and women (**B**) for the push-up test.

TABLE 7.4 • Fitness Categories for Push-up

Category	Age (yr)											
	15-19		20-29		30-39		40-49		50-59		60-69	
Sex	M	F	M	F	M	F	M	F	M	F	M	F
Excellent	≥39	≥33	≥36	≥30	≥30	≥27	≥25	≥24	≥21	≥21	≥18	≥17
Very good	29-38	25-32	29-35	21-29	22-29	20-26	17-24	15-23	13-20	11-20	11-17	12-16
Good	23-28	18-24	22-28	15-20	17-21	13-19	13-16	11-14	10-12	7-10	8-10	5-11
Fair	18-22	12-17	17-21	10-14	12-16	8-12	10-12	5-10	7-9	2-6	5-7	2-4
Poor	≤17	≤11	≤16	≤9	≤11	≤7	≤9	≤4	≤6	≤1	≤4	≤1

Reprinted with permission from the Canadian Society for Exercise Physiology. *CSEP Physical Activity Training for Health® (CSEP-PATH®) Resource Manual.* 2nd ed. 2019.

number of push-ups that can be completed without rest is used to evaluate muscular endurance. Interpretive norms are located in Table 7.4.

Bench press tests are also used to assess upper body muscular endurance, and these may include assessing the number of repetitions a person can perform at a certain percentage of 1-RM or body weight (*e.g.*, 70%). Box 7.6 provides instructions on how to conduct the YMCA submaximal bench press test. Norms for this test are found elsewhere (18).

Functional Fitness Chair Stand

The chair stand test provides a standardized method for assessing lower body muscular strength and endurance (19). The procedure for this test is provided in Box 7.7, and interpretative norms are located in Table 7.5. This test is primarily used in adults over the age of 60 years (19).

Box 7.6   Procedures for the YMCA Submaximal Bench Press Test

The test requires a 35-pound bar for women and a bar with weights totaling 80 pounds for men.

1. Position the client on the bench with both feet on the floor.
2. A spotter should hand the barbell to the client (hands shoulder width apart) and be available throughout the test to grasp the barbell when necessary. The test is started in the down position with the bar touching the chest.
3. Set a metronome to 60 beats per minute and have the client perform a contraction by lifting the bar to full extension with one beat and then lowering the bar to touch the chest with the next beat. The lifting cadence will produce 30 repetitions per minute.
4. The test continues until the client cannot complete a repetition on schedule with the cadence while using correct form. (Note: For highly fit subjects, an upper limit may need to be established.)

Box 7.7   Procedures for the Chair Stand Test

1. Place the chair against a wall where it will be stable.
2. Sit in the middle of the chair with feet flat on the floor, shoulder width apart, and back straight.
3. Cross your arms at the wrist and place them against your chest, where they should remain throughout the test.
4. On the command of "go," the participant rises to the full standing position, then sits back down again for the completion of one repetition.
5. The participant completes as many repetitions as possible in 30 seconds, without any use of the arms.

From Rikli RE, Jones CJ. Development and validation of a functional fitness test for community-residing older adults. *J Aging Phys Act.* 1999;7(2):129–161.

TABLE 7.5 • Categories for the Functional Fitness Chair Stand Test Age and Sex

| Category | Age (yr) | | | | | | | | | | | |
| | 60–64 | | 65–69 | | 70–74 | | 75–79 | | 80–84 | | 85–89 | |
Sex	M	W	M	W	M	W	M	W	M	W	M	W
Above Average	>19	>17	>18	>16	>17	>15	>17	>15	>15	>14	>14	>13
Average	14–19	12–17	12–18	11–16	12–17	10–15	11–17	10–15	10–15	9–14	8–14	8–13
Below Average	<14	<12	<12	<11	<12	<10	<11	<10	<10	<9	<8	<8

M, men; W, women.
Adapted, with permission, from R. E. Rikli and C. J. Jones, 2013, *Senior Fitness Test Manual*, 2nd ed. (Champaign, IL: Human Kinetics), 64, 89, 90.

Field Tests

Field tests are particularly useful when testing a large number of people at one time. In addition, field tests do not typically require any equipment and thus can be performed in many different locations, including at home. The two most common field tests are the push-up test and the curl-up test, each with different protocol options, some counting the number of repetitions completed in a fixed period of time and some counting the absolute number of repetitions completed. It is important to follow the proper procedures to establish the normative values that will be used for interpretation.

The push-up test is a popular field test, which was described earlier. The curl-up (crunch) test has been used historically as a measure of abdominal muscular endurance. However, most curl-up tests are moderately related to abdominal endurance ($r = 0.46$ to -0.50) and poorly related to abdominal strength ($r = -0.21$ to -0.36) (20,21). In addition, the benefits of this test as an assessment tool do not appear to exceed the potential risk of low back injury; thus, the curl-up test is no longer included in the *ACSM's Guidelines.*

INTERPRETATION ISSUES

There are several issues that make the interpretation muscular fitness assessments results difficult, including the different types of contractions, the possibility of a learning effect, improper positioning or incorrect form, and differences between various methods of loading the resistance. Owing to these multiple factors, a standardized assessment of muscular strength and/or muscular endurance has not been developed.

This chapter provides a variety of assessment procedures that have been used for many years and for which some normative data exist, which allow for interpretation of the muscular strength and muscular endurance of certain muscles. When using normative data, it is critical to follow the standardized test procedures, which include using the same equipment as was used by the population from which the norms were developed. This may be difficult when resistance exercise machines were used to develop norms, such as found in Table 7.3 for the leg press. The leg press data were developed from the Cooper Clinic, where all assessments were performed using the universal dynamic variable resistance (DVR) multistation resistance machines, which were widely available in fitness centers, gyms, and universities at the time. This highlights the dilemma when comparing and assessing participants tested with free weights or other brands of resistance exercise machines. Although ACSM continues to use this as the primary interpretation chart for this test with the presumption that the weight-to-press ratio will be similar using other equipment, caution must be exercised because this has not been objectively validated.

Another debated issue is whether to use absolute amounts of weight lifted or to make the amount of weight lifted a proportion of the participant's body weight. The norms developed for the bench press and leg press use the ratio method for interpreting results.

Owing to the limitations in having acceptable norms for interpretation, many fitness professionals opt to use baseline assessments of muscular strength and endurance as a reference point for a individual, for which future assessments will be compared. Although this does not allow an individual to know how he or she compares to others in the same age group or to a criterion-referenced standard, it does provide considerable information to develop a participant exercise program that allows for reliable assessments of progress over time.

SUMMARY

There are several established tests available to the exercise professional that can be used for the assessment of muscular fitness. Although unique factors exist that do not allow for one single measurement of either muscular strength or muscular endurance, there is considerable utility of the tests described in this chapter and therefore should be considered an important part of the assessments.

LABORATORY ACTIVITIES

Assessment of Muscular Strength

Data Collection

Work in groups of two or three. If you are working in a group of three, one person will be the subject, another the technician, and another the recorder. Rotate responsibilities until each person has had a chance to serve in each role. Collect the following data on one other member in your group. Record your values on your data sheet.

Handgrip dynamometer (kg):

	Right	Left
Trial 1		
Trial 2		
Trial 3		
Best score		Sum
Rating (Table 7.1)		

Upper body strength
   1-RM (lb)
   Body weight (lb)
   Bench press weight ratio
   Percentile ranking (Table 7.2)

Lower body strength
   1-RM (lb)
   Leg press weight ratio
   Percentile ranking (Table 7.3)

Laboratory Report

a. Describe your overall muscular strength based on these three measurements. Explain any limitations that apply to making this interpretation of overall muscular strength.

b. Locate a different set of norms for these three tests. How do the interpretations differ between the norms from the tables in this manual and the ones you found? Be sure to include the reference for the other set of norms.

Muscular Endurance Assessment

Data Collection

Work in groups of two or three. If you are working in a group of three, one person will be the participant, another the technician, and another the recorder. Rotate responsibilities until each person has had a chance to serve in each role. Collect the following data on one other member in your group. Record your values on your data sheet.

Push-ups: _____

Number of push-ups: _____

Percentile ranking (Table 7.5): _____

Laboratory Report

a. Describe your overall muscular endurance based on these measurements. Explain any limitations that apply to making this interpretation of overall muscular endurance.
b. Locate a different set of norms for these tests. How do the interpretations differ between the norms from the tables in this manual and the ones you found? Be sure to include the reference for the other set of norms.

REFERENCES

1. Garber CE, Blissmer B, Deschenes MR, et al.; American College of Sports Medicine Position Stand. Quantity and quality of exercise for developing and maintaining cardiorespiratory, musculoskeletal, and neuromotor fitness in apparently healthy adults: guidance for prescribing exercise. *Med Sci Sports Exerc*. 2011;43(7):1334–59. doi:10.1249/MSS.0b013e318213fefb.
2. US Department of Health and Human Services. *Physical Activity Guidelines for Americans*. 2nd ed. Washington (DC): Department of Health and Human Services; 2018. Available from: https://health.gov/paguidelines/second-edition/.
3. Gibson AL, Wagner DR, Heyward VH. *Principles of Assessment, Prescription, and Exercise Program Adherence. Advanced Fitness Assessment and Exercise Prescription*. 8th ed. Champaign: Human Kinetics; 2019. p. 56.
4. American College of Sports Medicine. *American College of Sports Medicine Position Stand. Progression models in resistance training for healthy adults. Med Sci Sports Exerc*. 2009;41(3):687–708. doi:10.1249/MSS.0b013e3181915670.
5. Reid KF, Fielding RA. Skeletal muscle power: a critical determinant of physical functioning in older adults. *Exerc Sport Sci Rev*. 2012;40(1):4–12. doi:10.1097/JES.0b013e31823b5f13.
6. Katula JA, Rejeski WJ, Marsh AP. Enhancing quality of life in older adults: a comparison of muscular strength and power training. *Health Qual Life Outcomes*. 2008;6:45. doi:10.1186/1477-7525-6-45.
7. Dodds RM, Syddall HE, Cooper R, et al. Grip strength across the life course: normative data from twelve British studies. *PLoS One*. 2014;9(12):e113637. doi:10.1371/journal.pone.0113637.
8. Dodds RM, Syddall HE, Cooper R, Kuh D, Cooper C, Sayer AA. Global variation in grip strength: a systematic review and meta-analysis of normative data. *Age Ageing*. 2016;45(2):209–16. doi:10.1093/ageing/afv192.
9. McGrath RP, Kraemer WJ, Snih SA, Peterson MD. Handgrip strength and health in aging adults. *Sports Med*. 2018;48(9):1993–2000. doi:10.1007/s40279-018-0952-y.
10. Shaughnessy KA, Hackney KJ, Clark BC, et al. A narrative review of handgrip strength and cognitive functioning: bringing a new characteristic to muscle memory. *J Alzheimers Dis*. 2020;73(4):1265–78. doi:10.3233/JAD-190856.
11. Wong SL. Grip strength reference values for Canadians aged 6 to 79: Canadian Health Measures Survey, 2007 to 2013. *Health Rep*. 2016;27(10):3–10.
12. Fernandez R. One repetition maximum clarified. *J Orthop Sports Phys Ther*. 2001;31(5):264.
13. Dohoney P, Chromiak JA, Lemire D, Abadie BR, Kovacs C. Prediction of one repetition maximum (1-RM) strength from a 4-6 RM and a 7-10 RM submaximal strength test in healthy young adult males. *J Exerc Physiol Online*. 2002;5(3):54–9.
14. Pereira MIR, Gomes PSC. Muscular strength and endurance tests: reliability and prediction of one repetition maximum–review and new evidences. *Rev Bras Med Esporte*. 2003;9(5):336–46.
15. Pérez-Castilla A, Jerez-Mayorga D, Martínez-García D, Rodríguez-Perea Á, Chirosa-Ríos LJ, García-Ramos A. Comparison of the bench press one-repetition maximum obtained by different procedures: direct assessment vs. lifts-to-failure equations vs. two-point method. *Int J Sports Sci Coaching*. 2020. doi:10.1177/1747954120911312.
16. Sheppard JM, Triplett NT. Program design for resistance training. In: Haff GG, Triplett NT, editors. *Essentials of Strength Training and Conditioning*. 4th ed. Champaign (IL): Human Kinetics; 2016. p. 439–469.
17. Logan P, Fornasiero D, Abernathy P. Protocols for the assessment of isoinertial strength. In: Gore CJ, editor. *Physiological Tests for Elite Athletes*. Champaign (IL): Human Kinetics; 2000. p. 200–221.
18. Golding LA. *YMCA Fitness Testing and Assessment Manual*. Champaign: Human Kinetics; 2000. p. 247.

19. Rikli RE, Jones CJ. Development and validation of a functional fitness test for community-residing older adults. *J Aging Phys Act.* 1999;7(2):129–61.

20. Knudson D, Johnston D. Validity and reliability of a bench trunk-curl test of abdominal endurance. *J Strength Cond Res.* 1995;9(3):165–9.

21. Knudson D. The validity of recent curl-up tests in young adults. *J Strength Cond Res.* 2001;15(1):81–5.

22. Canadian Society for Exercise Physiology. *Canadian Physical Activity, Fitness & Lifestyle Approach: CSEP—Health & Fitness Program's Health-Related Appraisal & Counselling Strategy.* Ottawa (ON): Canadian Society for Exercise Physiology; 2004.

23. Strand SL, Hjelm J, Shoepe, TC, et al. Norms for an isometric muscle endurance test. *J Hum Kinet.* 2014;40:93–102.

FLEXIBILITY

Flexibility is an important component of fitness because inadequate flexibility decreases the performance of activities of daily living. In addition, poor lower back and hip flexibility may contribute to the development of lower back pain (1,2), which is one of the more costly medical issues around the world (3).

Determining flexibility of specific joints yields valuable information to an overall fitness assessment. As with other measures, flexibility measures are useful as baseline measures to allow comparison of changes following a training program or serially over time as one ages. These baseline and periodic assessments can also identify joints with below desirable levels of flexibility, which can then be targeted for improvement in exercise training programs. In addition, these assessments may help in identifying bilateral strength imbalances in the muscles functioning about the joint. When assessing joint range of motion (ROM), bilateral comparison can identify differences in ROM between the left and right structures being evaluated. ROM deviations may lead to muscle imbalances and cause adjacent joint and muscle structures to overcompensate within the kinetic chain of movement, resulting in dysfunction within the related joint structures and the potential to develop injuries, trauma, and movement pattern complications.

UNIQUE ASSESSMENT PRINCIPLES

Flexibility is the functional capacity of the joints to move through a full ROM. The gold standard for determining flexibility is the laboratory assessment of the ROM of a specific joint. There are hundreds of joints in the human body, each of which can have a different level of flexibility; therefore, entire manuals have been devoted to assessment of ROM of the human body joints (4,5). Flexibility is joint specific and, therefore, will vary depending on which muscle and joint are being evaluated. This essentially rules out the possibility of a single test that can truly characterize one's flexibility. In addition, each joint has a set ROM that is unique to the function of the specific joint.

An adequate warm-up is essential before assessing flexibility. The warm-up should begin with some low-intensity whole-body aerobic exercise, such as walking or cycling. Ideally, both upper and lower body should be involved in the warm-up to increase whole-body blood flow and temperature. Some dynamic stretching and ROM exercises of the joints to be assessed should then follow the aerobic warm-up.

RANGE OF MOTION DEFINED

Many of the joints of the body can perform several different kinds of movements, in different planes and at different angles, depending on the type of joint structure and its designated function (5) (Figure 8.1). *Range of motion* (ROM) is defined as the range through which a joint can be moved, usually its range of flexion and extension, as determined by the type of joint, its articular surfaces, and that allowed by regional muscles, tendons, ligaments, joints, and physiologic control of movement across the joint (6). To measure ROM, it is recommended to start in the anatomical position — posture where the upper limbs are by the person's side and the palms of the hand are facing forward with fingers extended, whereas the lower limbs are together and facing forward (Figure 8.2). In the anatomic start position, the body is set at 0 degrees of flexion, extension, abduction, and adduction.

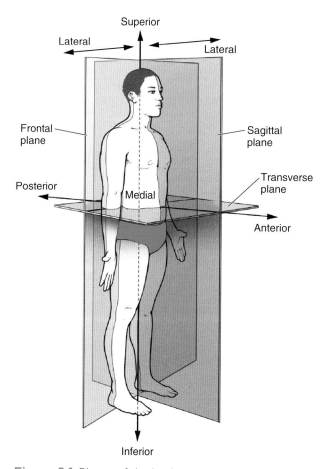

Figure 8.1 Planes of the body.

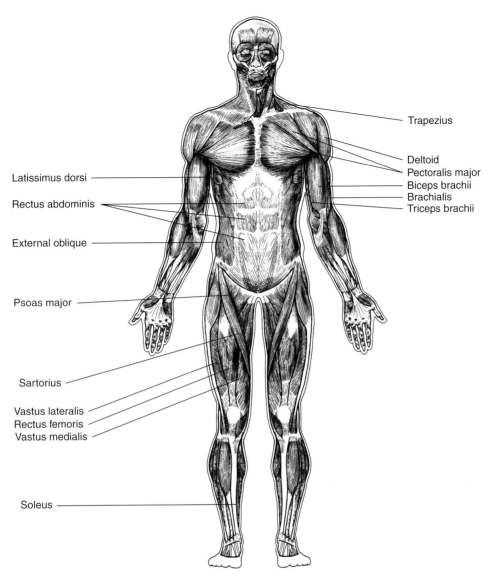

Figure 8.2 Anatomic start position.

ROM can be assessed either passively or actively. Passive ROM is the motion produced by the application of an external force, typically an examiner, without the assistance from the participant being tested. Conversely, active ROM is the area of motion achieved by the participant, as a result of voluntary contractions, without assistance by an examiner. Whereas passive ROM is typically performed by an exercise professional or allied health professionals (*e.g.*, physical therapists, athletic trainers, kinesiotherapists) for specific medical evaluations, the fitness professional will typically perform active ROM assessments to evaluate flexibility. Moreover, the fitness professional should be aware of several key factors known to influence flexibility in adults. Age (flexibility tends to decrease with age), sex (flexibility of specific joints is different), previous injuries to the joint (if structural damage occurred or if a surgical procedure was needed), and specific diseases that affect the joint (*e.g.*, arthritis) are all factors that may impact flexibility. In addition, five factors are significant to a joint structure's ROM:

1. The shape of the articular or bony surfaces between body segments
2. The structure of the joint, including ligaments, cartilage, bursae, fascia, and joint capsule
3. Structure of muscles and tendons
4. Joint disease such as chondromalacia, osteoarthritis, and bursitis
5. Neurological conditions such as cerebral palsy, stroke, and multiple sclerosis

It is worth noting that both hypomobility and hypermobility may be normal for a participant; however, these may also be the result of abnormalities of the joint surfaces, such as shortening of the joint capsule, ligaments, muscles, fascia, and skin. Therefore, some form of medical screening should be carried out before any flexibility assessment.

METHODS OF MEASUREMENT

Many different methods are used for assessing flexibility. These methods range from fairly simple visual methods, to measuring the change in reach distance, to using specially designed devices to assess ROM, including new technology that uses digital video cameras and software. The most widely used device for determining ROM is a goniometer, which is considered the gold-standard measure for flexibility assessment. Most goniometers are manually operated; however, those with an electronic scale can be used (electrogoniometers). Other common devices for assessing flexibility include the Leighton flexometer and inclinometers.

Goniometers: Tools to Measure Range of Motion

The specific joint ROM is measurable using an instrument known as a goniometer. Goniometry consists of assessment techniques that measure and compare the change in joint angles in degrees of motion (6). The goniometer comes in many different shapes (0–180 degrees or 0–360 degrees), sizes (length of the arms), and materials (metal or plastic). The design of the goniometer, as shown in Figure 8.3, includes the body (which includes the center axis, fulcrum, or center point), a stabilization arm, and a movement arm.

The body of a goniometer is similar to a protractor and consists of the arc of a circle. Around the circle are degree measurements that will range from 0 to 180 degrees or from 0 to 360 degrees, depending on the model. The axis or fulcrum is centered to the identified anatomic landmark required for a given ROM assessment. The stabilization arm establishes the starting position of the measurement. The movement arm is the body segment of the goniometer that will move in relation to the participant's movement during the test. The movement arm is set at the end position of the participants ROM.

Goniometry assessment is helpful in four important ways:

1. Provides immediate ROM feedback
2. Identifies muscle imbalances. When assessing joint ROM for a bilateral comparison, the goniometer may indicate differences in ROM between the left and right structures being evaluated. ROM deviations may lead to muscle imbalances and cause adjacent joint and muscle structures to overcompensate within the kinetic chain of movement, resulting in dysfunction within the related joint structures and the potential to develop injuries, trauma, and movement pattern complications.

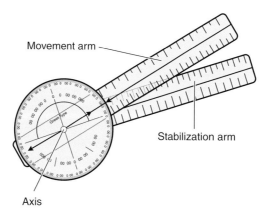

Figure 8.3 A goniometer, including the body axis or fulcrum, a stabilization arm, and a movement arm.

3. Identifies current ranges of motion before the exercise program starts. This assessment, in turn, provides a base of departure for the progress of the exercise program, specifically when implementing the flexibility and resistance components.

4. Provides baseline measurements from which plans can be made for future exercise goals. The first ROM test of primary joints necessary to future exercise movements indicates what can be achieved within time and schedule limitations.

RANGE OF MOTION ASSESSMENT

Before beginning any assessment, it is important the participant has provided consent, and at a minimum, a PAR-Q+ has been provided as a screening tool. Moreover, before the assessment, the participant should be given appropriate time to warm up. Before starting any movement, the participant should be provided a demonstration of the ROM test to be performed and explain the assessment process. As each joint's ROM is assessed, the proper starting position, performance of the ROM test, and ending position should all be demonstrated. Instructions of how to use a goniometer for measurement of a joint is provided in Box 8.1.

In all ROM assessments, location of the goniometer for the fulcrum, stabilization arm, and movement arm need to be clearly specified to ensure accurate measurements.

Before the assessment begins, provide the participant with an overview of the goniometry process and the purpose of the assessment. A demonstration of a sample ROM test on a joint to explain how the assessment works precedes the actual assessment. As each joint's ROM is assessed, demonstrate the proper starting position, performance of the ROM test, and the ending position. The following process needs to be completed first to attain the starting measurement:

● Participant needs to assume optimal posture in most goniometry assessments.
● Participant's joint structure is in 0 degrees starting position.
● Special starting position considerations are identified under specific joint ROM tests explained later in this chapter.
● The goniometer starts at the joint axis or hinge point where the axis of rotation occurs for the two body segments.
● The goniometer's stabilization and movement arms are centered along each body segment.

Move the body segment slowly through the ROM as instructed. Remind the participant that the assessment is not a competition, and as soon as the body segment cannot move further without

---

Box 8.1 Goniometer Assessment

The following processes describe the position of the goniometer (10):

● Identify anatomical landmark and joint axis.
● Stabilize the body part proper alignment from the start to ending positions.
● Locate the fulcrum at the joint axis or hinge point where the axis of rotation occurs for the two body segments involved.
● Place the stabilization and movement arms so that they are centered along each body segment according to the landmarks for each joint measurement. (Note that the goniometer arms should be long enough to properly align with the landmarks.)
● The stabilization arm of the goniometer will need to remain stationary, whereas the movement arm moves with the body segment through the ROM.
● With the goniometer aligned to the specific body segment, the participant should be instructed to actively move the body segment slowly through the ROM until the body segment cannot move further without causing discomfort or shifting other body parts. When there is no further movement, the angle between the stabilization and movements arms (joint angle) is measured and recorded.
● Measurement is read and recorded correctly.
● Careful observations are made whether each joint's ROM assessment is pain free.

compensating the body through shifting or pushing beyond the ROM, stop the movement. Stress that the movement of the given body segment is slow through its ROM. One arm of the goniometer needs to be stabilized, while the other arm moves with the second body segment until the body segment stops. When there is no further movement, the joint angle is then measured and recorded. The use of goniometry can be an accurate measure of a joint's ROM when the following procedures are properly performed (7):

- All anatomical landmarks are identified.
- The joint axis point has been clearly defined.
- Stabilize the body in proper alignment from the start to ending positions.
- Instruct the participant to move slowly through the proper ROM, and keep the goniometer aligned to each body segment.
- Read and record measurements correctly.
- Be familiar with the normal ROM for each joint structure.
- Observe whether each joint's ROM assessment is pain free.

In addition, stabilization of surrounding body parts must occur, and starting and ending body positions must be defined and measured precisely. In the following section are specifications for the various ROM assessments of the back, shoulder, and hip. An average ROM for each assessment is also provided in Table 8.1.

This chapter focuses on the assessment of some of the major joints in the body that are used to perform physical activities and exercise for health-related reasons. Assessments made with measures of reach distance and with a goniometer are both reviewed.

JOINT MOVEMENTS

The ROM assessments provided below focus on primary joint and muscle structures essential to exercise program design. These goniometry assessments are not a complete list of all the possible joint movements that could be measured.

TABLE 8.1 • Range of Motion of Select Single Joint Movements in Degrees

	Degrees		Degrees
Shoulder girdle movement			
Flexion	90–120	Extension	20–60
Abduction	80–100		
Horizontal abduction	30–45	Horizontal adduction	90–135
Medial rotation	70–90	Lateral rotation	70–90
Elbow movement			
Flexion	135–160		
Supination	75–90	Pronation	75–90
Trunk movement			
Flexion	120–150	Extension	20–45
Lateral flexion	10–35	Rotation	20–40
Hip movement			
Flexion	90–135	Extension	10–30
Abduction	30–50	Adduction	10–30
Medial rotation	30–45	Lateral rotation	45–60
Knee movement			
Flexion	130–140	Extension	5–10
Ankle movement			
Dorsiflexion	15–20	Plantar flexion	30–50
Inversion	10–30	Eversion	10–20

Adapted from Levangie PK, Norkin CC, Lewek MD. *Joint Structure and Function.* 6th ed. Philadelphia (PA): F.A. Davis; 2019. p. 552.

The Neck

Cervical Flexion

The plane of motion: sagittal
The axis of motion: coronal/frontal
Average range: 0 to 45 degrees

Goniometer position:

1. Axis point: external auditory meatus
2. Stabilization arm: perpendicular to the floor
3. Movement arm: parallel to the floor; midline of goniometer is level with the inferior bottom of the nose.

Stabilization: Participant is in good posture with a stabilized scapula and thoracic and lumbar spine.
Starting/ending body position: Participant is seated with cervical spine in 0 degrees of flexion, extension, rotation, or lateral flexion. Head is in neutral position. Participant performs cervical flexion until the first sign of resistance (Figure 8.4B).

Cervical Extension

The plane of motion: sagittal
The axis of motion: coronal/frontal
Average range: 0 to 45 degrees

Goniometer position:

1. Axis point: external auditory meatus
2. Stabilization arm: perpendicular to the floor
3. Movement arm: parallel to the floor; midline of goniometer is level with the inferior bottom of the nose.

Stabilization: Participant is in good posture with a stabilized scapula and thoracic and lumbar spine.
Starting/ending body position: Participant is seated with cervical spine in 0 degrees of flexion, extension, rotation, or lateral flexion. Head is in neutral position. Participant performs cervical extension until the first sign of resistance (Figure 8.4C).

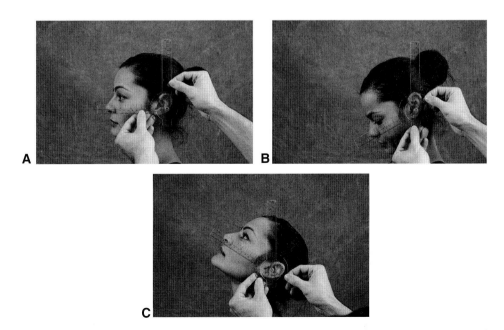

Figure 8.4 Assessment of cervical flexion and cervical extension. **A:** Baseline. **B:** Cervical flexion. **C:** Cervical extension.

Lateral Flexion

> The plane of motion: frontal
> The axis of motion: anterior/posterior
> Average range: 0 to 45 degrees

Goniometer position:

1. Axis point: cervical 7
2. Stabilization arm: perpendicular to the floor
3. Movement arm: midline of the head; occipital protuberance for reference

Stabilization: Participant is in good posture with a stabilized scapula and thoracic and lumbar spine.

Starting/ending body position: Participant is seated with cervical spine in 0 degrees of flexion, extension, rotation, or lateral flexion. Head is in neutral position. Participant performs lateral flexion until the first sign of resistance (Figure 8.5).

Lumbar Spine

Unlike other structures in the body, to assess ROM of the lumbar (back) section, a tape measure is recommended. The tape measure should be in contact with the participant's spine throughout the measure.

Lumbar Flexion

To assess lumbar flexion, tape is positioned with the zero mark at the spinous process C7, and measurement is taken down to the superior iliac (or level to the posterior superior iliac spine [PSIS]; Figure 8.6). The participant performs lumbar flexion until the first sign of resistance, and the increase in distance is recorded. An average range for healthy adults is a 4-in increase as the spine flexes.

> The plane of motion: sagittal
> The axis of motion: coronal/frontal
> Average range: 4-in increase

Tape measure position:

1. Top point: spinous processes C7
2. Bottom point: S1 or level to PSIS

Stabilization: Participant seated on floor or table with pelvis stabilized to prevent anterior/posterior tilting with legs extended.

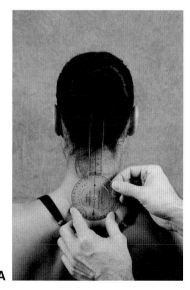 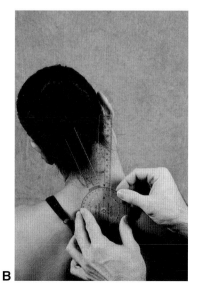

Figure 8.5 Assessment of cervical lateral flexion. **A:** Baseline position. **B:** Lateral flexion.

Starting/ending body position: Participant is in good posture with a stabilized cervical, thoracic, and lumbar spine in 0 degree of flexion, extension, rotation, or lateral flexion. Head is in neutral position. Participant performs lumbar flexion until the first sign of resistance (Figure 8.6B).

Lumbar Extension

To assess lumbar extension, tape is positioned with the zero mark at the spinous process C7, and measurement is taken down to the superior iliac (or level to the PSIS; Figure 8.6). The participant performs lumbar extension until the first sign of resistance. An average range for healthy adults is a 2-in increase as the spine extends.

The plane of motion: sagittal
The axis of motion: coronal/frontal
Average range: 2 in difference as spine extends

Tape measure position:

1. Top point: spinous processes C7
2. Bottom point: S1 or level to PSIS

Stabilization: Participant seated on floor or table with pelvis stabilized to prevent anterior/posterior tilting with legs extended.

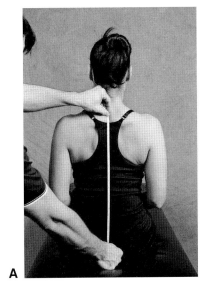
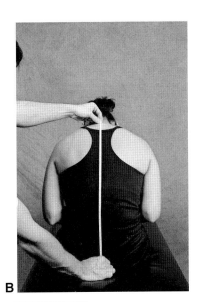
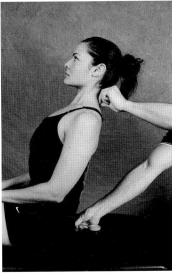

Figure 8.6 Assessment of lumbar flexion and lumbar extension. **A:** Baseline position. **B:** Lumbar flexion. **C:** Lumbar extension.

Starting/ending body position: Participant is in good posture with a stabilized cervical, thoracic, and lumbar spine in 0 degrees of flexion, extension, rotation, or lateral flexion. Head is in neutral position. Participant performs lumbar extension until the first sign of resistance (Figure 8.6C).

Finger to Floor Method

A quicker method to examine flexion of the spine is the finger to floor method. Unlike the methods described earlier, in this method, the measurement is not done over the lumbar spine; instead, the measurement is done between the participant's fingers and the floor using a measuring tape (7) or yard stick (8).

To assess lumbar spine using the finger to floor method, the participant is asked to simply bend forward and stretch their arms toward the floor while maintaining the knees, arms, and fingers fully extended; the distance between the tip of the middle finger and the floor is measured with a tape measure (Figure 8.7). A modified version of the test has also been validated (9), where the participant stands on a stool (32.4 cm high) and bends forward toward the floor. In this case, measurements of the distances above the stool were positive and those below the stool were negative. A zero was recorded if the patient reached the top of the stool.

Even though standard values for the finger to floor method do not exist, several ranges are provided in the literature. Improvements in lumbar flexion, however, can be assessed with shortening the distance between the hands and the floor, or a decrease in pain as the person moves through flexion, following a well-designed exercise program for the back.

The Shoulder (Glenohumeral Joint)

Glenohumeral Flexion

The plane of motion: sagittal
The axis of motion: coronal/frontal
Average range: 0 to 90 degrees

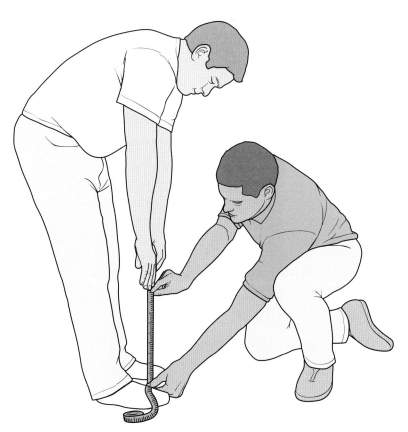

Figure 8.7 Assessment of lumbar flexion using the finger to floor method.

Goniometer position:

1. Axis point: lateral aspect of greater tubercle
2. Stabilization arm: perpendicular to the floor
3. Movement arm: aligned with midline of humerus and referenced with the lateral epicondyle

Stabilization: Participant is in good posture with a stabilized thoracic and lumbar spine. With a retracted scapula, stabilize the scapula to prevent tilting, rotation, or elevation.

Starting/ending body position: With the participant either standing or seated and with the glenohumeral joint in 0 degrees of flexion, extension, abduction, or adduction. Head is in neutral position. Palm of hand should face the body. Elbow should be extended completely. Participant performs glenohumeral flexion until the first sign of resistance (Figure 8.8). (Note that this can also be performed with participant starting in supine position, with hips and knees flexed.)

Glenohumeral Extension

The plane of motion: sagittal
The axis of motion: coronal/frontal
Average range: 0 to 60 degrees

Goniometer position:

1. Axis point: lateral aspect of greater tubercle
2. Stabilization arm: parallel to the floor
3. Movement arm: aligned with midline of the lateral humerus and referenced with the lateral epicondyle

Stabilization: Participant is in good posture with a stabilized thoracic and lumbar spine. With a retracted scapula, stabilize the scapula to prevent tilting, rotation, or elevation. Place towel under humerus to stabilize and align with acromion process.

Starting/ending body position: Participant is prone on the table with glenohumeral in 0 degrees of flexion, extension, abduction, or adduction. Head is in neutral position. Palm of hand should face the body. Elbow should be extended completely. Participant performs glenohumeral extension until the first sign of resistance (Figure 8.9).

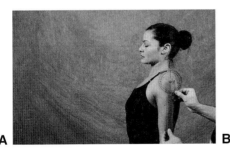
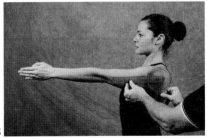

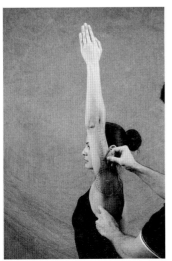

Figure 8.8 Assessment of shoulder flexion range of motion. **A:** Baseline position. **B:** Partial shoulder flexion. **C:** Full shoulder flexion.

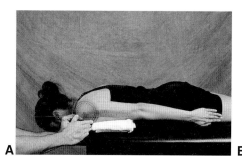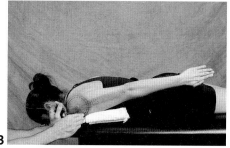

Figure 8.9 Assessment of shoulder extension range of motion. **A:** Baseline position. **B:** Shoulder extension.

Glenohumeral Adduction (Palm Facing Body)

The plane of motion: frontal
The axis of motion: anterior/posterior
Average range: 0 to 180 degrees

Goniometer position:

1. Axis point: 1 in distal to the acromion process at the posterior shoulder
2. Stabilization arm: perpendicular to the floor
3. Movement arm: align with midline of posterior humerus and reference the olecranon process of the elbow

Stabilization: Participant is in good posture with a stabilized scapula (retracted) and thoracic and lumbar spine. Stabilize scapula to prevent tilting, rotation, or elevation.

Starting/ending body position: Participant is seated with arm extended perpendicular to the body. Head is in neutral position. Palm of hand should be facing the body. With arm extended, participant performs glenohumeral adduction (move arms toward the body) until the first sign of resistance.

Glenohumeral Abduction (Palm Facing Away from Body)

The plane of motion: frontal
The axis of motion: anterior/posterior
Average range: 0 to 180 degrees

Goniometer position:

1. Axis point: 1 in distal to the acromion process at the posterior shoulder
2. Stabilization arm: perpendicular to the floor
3. Movement arm: align with midline of posterior humerus and reference the olecranon process of the elbow

Stabilization: Participant is in good posture with a stabilized scapula (retracted) and thoracic and lumbar spine. Stabilize scapula to prevent tilting, rotation, or elevation.

Starting/ending body position: Participant is seated with arm extended parallel to the body. Head is in neutral position. Palm of hand should be facing the body. With arm extended, participant performs glenohumeral abduction (moves arm away from the body) until the first sign of resistance.

Glenohumeral Internal Rotation

The plane of motion: transverse
The axis of motion: longitudinal
Average range: 0 to 70 degrees

Goniometer position:

1. Axis point: olecranon process of the elbow
2. Stabilization arm: perpendicular to the floor
3. Movement arm: align with lateral midline of ulna and reference the ulnar styloid

Baseline

Internal rotation

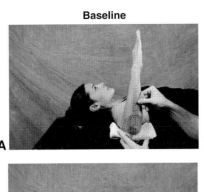

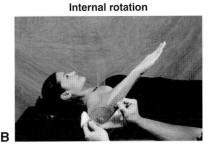

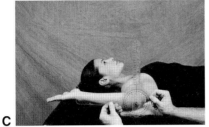

External rotation

Figure 8.10 Assessment of shoulder rotation. **A:** Baseline position. **B:** Internal shoulder rotation. **C:** External shoulder rotation.

Stabilization: Participant is in good posture with a stabilized scapula (retracted) and thoracic and lumbar spine. Stabilize scapula to prevent tilting, rotation, or elevation. Place towel under humerus to stabilize and align with acromion process.

Starting/ending body position: Participant is supine on table with humerus abducted at 90 degrees and elbow is flexed at 90 degrees. Elbow is at 0 degrees of supination and pronation. Participant performs glenohumeral internal rotation until the first sign of resistance (Figure 8.10B).

Glenohumeral External Rotation

The plane of motion: transverse
The axis of motion: longitudinal
Average range: 0 to 90 degrees

Goniometer position:

1. Axis point: olecranon process of the elbow
2. Stabilization arm: perpendicular to the floor
3. Movement arm: align with lateral midline of ulna and reference the ulnar styloid

Stabilization: Participant is in good posture with a stabilized scapula (retracted) and thoracic and lumbar spine. Stabilize scapula to prevent tilting, rotation, or elevation. Place towel under humerus to stabilize and align with acromion process.

Starting/ending body position: Participant is supine on table, with humerus abducted at 90 degrees and elbow is flexed at 90 degrees. Elbow is at 0 degrees of supination and pronation. Participant performs glenohumeral external rotation until the first sign of resistance (Figure 8.10C).

The Hip (Acetabulofemoral Joint)

Flexion (Testing Leg Fully Extended)

The plane of motion: sagittal
The axis of motion: coronal/Frontal
Average range: 0 to 90 degrees

Goniometer position:

1. Axis point: greater trochanter of the lateral thigh
2. Stabilization arm: lateral midline of the pelvis
3. Movement arm: lateral midline of the femur, using the lateral epicondyle as a reference

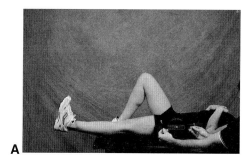

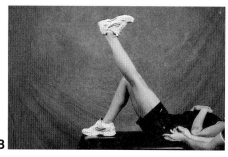

Figure 8.11 Assessment of hip flexion with leg fully extended. **A:** Baseline position. **B:** Hip flexion.

Stabilization: Participant is in good posture with a stabilized scapula, thoracic and lumbar spine, and pelvic area. Pelvis should not rise off table. Opposite leg not being assessed should have knee flexed and foot flat on table for added stability and protection for the back.

Starting/ending body position: Participant is supine on the table, with testing leg in 0 degrees of hip flexion and opposite knee in 90 degrees of flexion (the knee is flexed to reduce contraction of hamstrings). Participant performs hip flexion until the first sign of resistance or until the pelvis rotates or knee breaks extension (Figure 8.11).

Flexion (Testing Knee Flexed 90 Degrees and Hip Flexed 90 Degrees)

The plane of motion: sagittal
The axis of motion: coronal/frontal
Average range: 0 to 120 degrees

Goniometer position:

1. Axis point: greater trochanter of the lateral thigh
2. Stabilization arm: lateral midline of the pelvis
3. Movement arm: lateral midline of the femur, using the lateral epicondyle as a reference

Stabilization: Participant is in good posture with a stabilized scapula, thoracic and lumbar spine, and pelvic area. Pelvis should not rise off table. Opposite leg not being assessed should have knee extended on table for added stability and protection for the back.

Starting/ending body position: Participant is supine on table, with knee flexed at 90 degrees and hip flexed at 90 degrees; and hip is in 0 degrees of abduction, adduction, and rotation. Knee is flexed to reduce contraction of hamstrings. Participant performs hip flexion until the first sign of resistance or until the pelvis rotates (Figure 8.12).

Hip Extension (Testing Leg Fully Extended)

The plane of motion: sagittal
The axis of motion: coronal/frontal
Average range: 0 to 30 degrees

Goniometer position:

1. Axis point: greater trochanter of the lateral thigh
2. Stabilization arm: lateral midline of the pelvis
3. Movement arm: lateral midline of the femur, using the lateral epicondyle as a reference

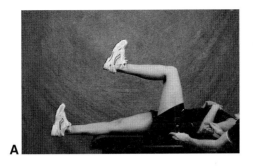

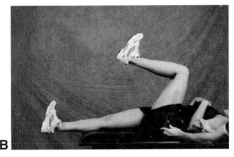

Figure 8.12 Assessment of hip flexion with testing knee and hip flexed 90 degrees. **A:** Baseline position. **B:** Hip flexion.

Stabilization: Participant is in good posture with a stabilized scapula, thoracic and lumbar spine, and pelvic area. Pelvis should not rise off the table. Opposite leg not being assessed should have leg fully extended on the table for added stability.

Starting/ending body position: Participant is prone on the table, with hip in 0 degrees of flexion, extension, abduction, adduction, and rotation. Testing leg has knee fully extended. Participant performs hip extension until the first sign of resistance or until the pelvis rotates (Figure 8.13).

Hip Abduction

The plane of motion: frontal
The axis of motion: anterior/posterior
Average range: 0 to 45 degrees

Goniometer position:

1. Axis point: locate at the anterior superior iliac spine (ASIS)
2. Stabilization arm: imaginary horizontal line connecting axis point ASIS to the other ASIS
3. Movement arm: anterior midline of the femur, using the midline of the patella as a reference

Stabilization: Participant is in good posture with a stabilized scapula, thoracic and lumbar spine, and pelvic area. Stabilize for lateral trunk flexion on both sides.

Starting/ending body position: Participant is supine on the table, with hip in 0 degrees of flexion, extension, and rotation. Arms should be crossed or away from legs. Testing leg has knee fully extended. Participant performs hip abduction until the first sign of resistance or lateral trunk flexion occurs on either side (Figure 8.14).

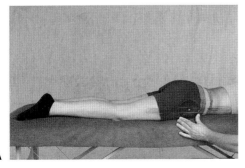
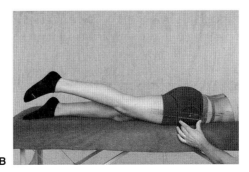

Figure 8.13 Hip extension range of motion. **A:** Baseline position. **B:** Hip extension.

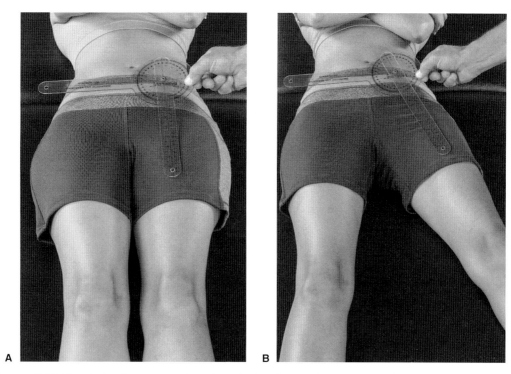

Figure 8.14 Hip abduction range of motion. **A:** Baseline position. **B:** Hip abduction.

Hip Adduction

The plane of motion: frontal
The axis of motion: anterior/posterior
Average range: 0 to 30 degrees

Goniometer position:

1. Axis point: located at the ASIS
2. Stabilization arm: imaginary horizontal line connecting axis point ASIS to the other ASIS
3. Movement arm: anterior midline of the femur, using the midline of the patella as a reference

Stabilization: Participant is in good posture with a stabilized scapula, thoracic and lumbar spine, and pelvic area. Opposite leg not being tested should be abducted fully to allow for testing hip to be assessed.

Starting/ending body position: Participant is supine on the table, with hip in 0 degrees of flexion, extension, and rotation. Testing leg has knee fully extended. Participant performs hip adduction until the first sign of resistance or lateral trunk flexion or pelvic rotation occurs (Figure 8.15).

INTERPRETATION

Reference ranges for ROM measurements are provided in Table 8.1. There are no universally accepted standards for ROM; thus, it is quite possible that some facilities or programs may use alternate reference ranges.

It is important to recognize that a learning effect is likely with flexibility measurements. A recommendation from the American Medical Association (1) suggests that ROM should be measured using three consecutive trials and averaged as the true value. If the average ROM is <50 degrees, three of the measurements must fall within ±5 degrees of the mean. If the average is ≥50 degrees, three measurements must fall within ±10 degrees of average. Such measures may be taken up to six times until they meet the criteria; otherwise, they are considered invalid.

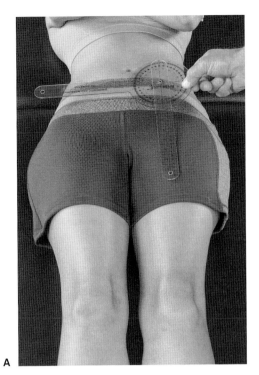 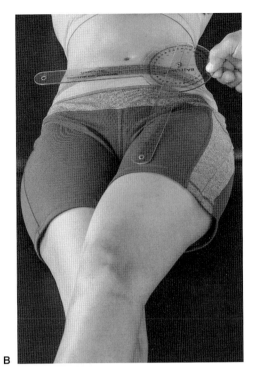

Figure 8.15 Hip adduction range of motion. **A:** Baseline position. **B:** Hip adduction.

SUMMARY

Similar to the muscular endurance assessment, there is no one single measurement that provides an overall measurement of flexibility. Fortunately, goniometer assessments are feasible and provide a reliable measurement of joint-specific flexibility. This assessment can provide valuable information to the fitness professional on how to design an effective exercise program, including flexibility exercises that would enhance the participant's flexibility.

LABORATORY ACTIVITIES

Range of Motion Assessments

Data Collection

Work with one other student (he or she measures you, you measure him or her) to perform the following ROM assessments. The measure is taken passively because the movement is slowly and gradually performed until maximum range is achieved as evidenced by high mechanical resistance or the discomfort of the participant.

Movement	Measure (Degrees)	
Neck		
Cervical flexion		
Cervical extension		
Lateral flexion		
Lumbar spine		
Lumbar flexion		
Lumbar extension		
Finger to floor method		

	Right	Left
The shoulder (glenohumeral joint)		
Glenohumeral flexion		
Glenohumeral extension		
Glenohumeral adduction (palm facing body)		
Glenohumeral abduction (palm facing away from body)		
Glenohumeral internal rotation		
Glenohumeral external rotation		
The hip (acetabulofemoral joint)		
Flexion (testing leg fully extended)		
Flexion (testing knee flexed 90 degrees and hip flexed 90 degrees)		
Hip extension (testing leg fully extended)		
Hip abduction		
Hip adduction		

Written Report

Provide an interpretation of your ROM for each measured movement. Highlight any results that were not within the expected average range for each measure. Were there any imbalances between assessments on the right versus the left side of the body? Comment on what problems could arise from poor flexibility test scores from these measurements.

Distance Tests for Flexibility Assessment

Data Collection

Work with one other student (he or she measures you, you measure him or her) to perform the following flexibility assessments. The measure is taken passively because the movement is slow and gradually performed until maximum range is achieved as evidenced by high mechanical resistance or the discomfort of the participant.

Lumbar flexion

Trial 1: _____   Trial 2: _____   Trial 3: _____   Best score: _____

Lumbar extension

Trial 1: _____   Trial 2: _____   Trial 3: _____   Best score: _____

Finger to Floor Test

Trial 1: _____   Trial 2: _____   Trial 3: _____   Best score: _____

Modified Finger to Floor Test

Trial 1: _____   Trial 2: _____   Trial 3: _____   Best score: _____

Written Report

Provide an interpretation of your flexibility for each test. Comment on what problems could arise from poor flexibility test scores from these measurements.

REFERENCES

1. Sadler SG, Spink MJ, Ho A, De Jonge XJ, Chuter VH. Restriction in lateral bending range of motion, lumbar lordosis, and hamstring flexibility predicts the development of low back pain: a systematic review of prospective cohort studies. *BMC Musculoskelet Disord.* 2017;18(1):179. doi:10.1186/s12891-017-1534-0.
2. Victora Ruas C, Vieira A. Do muscle strength imbalances and low flexibility levels lead to low back pain? A brief review. *J Funct Morphol Kinesiol.* 2017;2(3):29.
3. Mutubuki EN, Beljon Y, Maas ET, et al. The longitudinal relationships between pain severity and disability versus health-related quality of life and costs among chronic low back pain patients. *Qual Life Res.* 2020;29(1):275-87. doi:10.1007/s11136-019-02302-w.
4. Clarkson HM. *Musculoskeletal Assessment: Joint Motion and Muscle Testing.* Philadelphia (PA): Wolters Kluwer/Lippincott Williams & Wilkins Health; 2012.
5. Norkin CC, White DJ. *Measurement of Joint Motion: A Guide to Goniometry.* Philadelphia (PA): F.A. Davis Company; 2016.
6. Norkin CC, White DJ. Basic concepts. In: Norkin CC, White DJ, editors. *Measurement of Joint Motion: A Guide to Goniometry.* 5th ed. Philadelphia (PA): F.A. Davis Company; 2016.
7. Frost M, Stuckey S, Smalley LA, Dorman G. Reliability of measuring trunk motions in centimeters. *Phys Ther.* 1982;62(10):1431-7. doi:10.1093/ptj/62.10.1431.
8. Broer MR, Galles NR. Importance of relationship between various body measurements in performance of the toe-touch test. Research quarterly American Association for Health. *Phys Educ Recreation.* 1958;29(3):253-63.
9. Gauvin MG, Riddle DL, Rothstein JM. Reliability of clinical measurements of forward bending using the modified fingertip-to-floor method. *Phys Ther.* 1990;70(7):443-7. doi:10.1093/ptj/70.7.443.
10. Levangie PK, Norkin CC, Lewek MD. *Joint Structure and Function.* 6th ed. Philadelphia (PA): F.A. Davis Company; 2019. 552 p.

Electrocardiography

INTRODUCTION

Electrocardiography is the clinical representation and study of the electrical activity of the heart muscle (*i.e.*, myocardium). An electrocardiogram (abbreviated ECG or EKG, from the German "kardio") is a recording of the electrical activity of the heart. The ECG is one of the most basic and commonly used tools in diagnostic cardiology. Although helpful to diagnose heart disease, it is important to carefully evaluate and interpret ECGs, regardless of health status, as healthy individuals can also have abnormal ECGs.

The ECG provides information about rate, rhythm, and impulse conduction through the myocardium; pathology of the myocardium; previous heart disease and/or damage; and current physiologic status of the myocardium. Although a valuable tool for the diagnosis of cardiovascular disease (CVD), the development of more advanced techniques (*i.e.*, nuclear or echocardiographic imaging) has resulted in less reliance of the ECG as diagnostic tool.

Taking into account that depolarization of myocardial cells is normally a very orderly process, the *normal* ECG is consistent and relatively easy to discern because there are predictable waveforms as well as established normal time intervals for those waveforms. Abnormalities of myocardial anatomy and physiology, various CVDs, and many other influences can result in abnormal waveforms and/or rhythms. The normal ECG is discussed in this chapter.

CONDUCTION SYSTEM OF THE HEART

The anatomy of the conduction system is depicted in Figure 9.1. Electrical depolarization originates in the sinoatrial (SA) node, located in the right atrium near the superior vena cava. The wave of depolarization subsequently spreads through the right atrium into the left atrium and to the atrioventricular (AV) node. The impulse next proceeds through the AV node and depolarizes the bundle of His, which extends into the intraventricular septum, then into the right and left bundle branches. The right bundle branch travels down the right side of the septum and into the right ventricle (RV). The left bundle branch divides into anterior and posterior branches as it proceeds through the left ventricle (LV). The bundle branches terminate in Purkinje fibers, which are diffuse throughout the LV.

Table 9.1 presents the ECG wave associated with the corresponding electrical event in the myocardium.

The SA node is responsible for initiating depolarization of the myocardium. However, individuals with both normal and abnormal hearts may experience abnormal depolarization sequences. These abnormalities result in dysrhythmias and/or blocks that impact the ECG rhythm. The reader is referred to more advanced texts (1,2) as dysrhythmias and blocks are beyond the scope of this text.

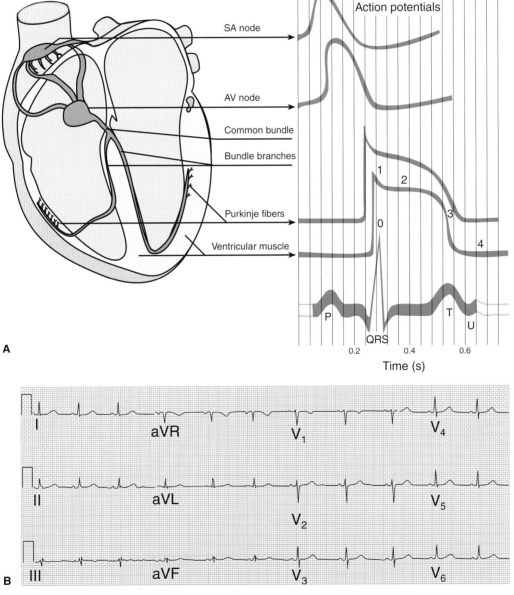

Figure 9.1 A: The electrical conduction of the heart and its relation to the ECG. **B:** Normal 12-lead ECG tracing. AV, atrioventricular; SA, sinoatrial. Source: Reprinted from Stouffer G, Runge MS, Patterson C, Rossi JS, editors. *Netter's Cardiology*. Philadelphia (PA): Elsevier; 2019.

TABLE 9.1 • Normal Sequence of Depolarization and the Electrocardiographic Correlation	
Sinoatrial node	Flat
Atrial depolarization	P wave
Atrioventricular node	PR interval
Bundle of His	PR interval
Purkinje fibers	PR interval
Ventricular muscle depolarization	QRS complex
Ventricular isoelectric period	ST segment
Ventricular muscle repolarization	T wave

BASICS

The Electrocardiogram Paper

Figure 9.2 shows the paper typically used to record the ECG. This paper is designed with a grid pattern consisting of thin and thick lines. The horizontal axis depicts time intervals in milliseconds (ms), whereas the vertical axis measures voltage in millivolts (mV). The thin lines are 1-mm marks lined horizontally (x-axis) and vertically (y-axis). The thicker lines are positioned every 5 mm.

In normally calibrated ECG paper, which is set at 25 mm $\cdot$ s^{-1}, each 1 mm in the horizontal axis represents 40 ms (0.04 seconds) of elapsed time. Thus, five "small" (1 mm) boxes equate to one "big" (5 mm) box, equivalent to 200 ms (0.20 seconds) (*e.g.*, 0.04 seconds $\times$ 5 = 0.20 seconds). On the vertical axis, each 1 mm represents 0.1 mV of voltage, where a 10-mm upward deflection includes 10 "little" or two "big" boxes, equivalent to 1 mV (10 small boxes $\times$ 0.1 mV). In the vertical axis, all deflections are measured from the isoelectric line, which is considered the baseline of the ECG. Deflections can be either positive or negative depending on the location of the electrode. By convention, upward deflections are referred to as *positive deflections*, and those moving downward are called *negative deflections*.

Equipment

All equipment used in both resting and exercise electrocardiography must be maintained and calibrated on a regular basis. Ongoing maintenance of such equipment should include electronic and mechanical checks by qualified biomedical engineers or technicians. ECG equipment is standardized with respect to paper speed and waveform deflection, and normally, the documentation of this standardization should be part of the warm-up routines on all ECG equipment. Treadmill calibration with respect to both speed and elevation should be checked on a regular basis. Other equipment used in both exercise

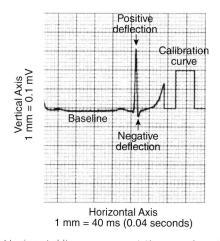

Figure 9.2 The ECG paper. Horizontal lines represent time, and vertical lines represent amplitude. Each horizontal "thin" line equals 1 mm (0.04 seconds), and each "thick" line equals 5 mm (0.20 seconds). The calibration box is 10 mm tall (1.0 mV). Source: Reprinted from Thompson WR, editor. *ACSM's Clinical Exercise Physiology*. Philadelphia (PA): Wolters Kluwer; 2018.

and resting electrocardiography must be regularly maintained and checked at least quarterly. All such quality checks must be documented, and records must be retained. Equipment that does not meet standards and that cannot be brought to standard calibration and operation should be discarded.

Waves, Segments, and Intervals

In a normal heart, the electrical activity begins in the atria (Figure 9.3). Thus, the cardiac cycle begins with depolarization of the SA node and spreads through the atria. Because the atria are small, thin-walled chambers, the deflections on the ECG will typically show smaller waveforms, known as the *P wave* (Figure 9.4). The normal P wave should be short in duration (<120 ms) and amplitude (<0.25 mV). The normal ranges for ECG parameters are listed in Box 9.1.

Following depolarization of the atria, a pause occurs before the electrical impulse reaches the ventricle. This pause is known as the *PR interval* (Figure 9.4). The PR interval begins at the beginning of the P wave and ends at the beginning of the QRS complex. A normal PR interval is between 120 and 200 ms (0.12–0.20 seconds) and is equivalent to three to five of the small boxes. Even though the PR interval is typically measured in Lead II, it can also be seen in other leads, such as in a 12-lead ECG.

Depolarization of the ventricles normally occurs after atrial depolarization. Ventricular depolarization in the ECG is depicted by the QRS complex, which should be short in length (≤100 ms or ≤0.10 seconds) and tall in amplitude (Figure 9.4). Although often referred to a single waveform, the QRS complex consists of three distinct deflections: a downward (negative) deflection called a *Q wave*, an upward (positive) deflection called an *R wave*, and a deflection returning to baseline called an *S wave*. Several deviations of the normal QRS pattern exist depending on disease or cardiac injury and are beyond the scope of this text.

The QRS is measured at the initial deflection of the QRS, weather it is negative (Q wave) or positive (R wave). The end point for the QRS is the end of the S wave if an S wave is present or the end of the R wave if an S wave is not present.

The last wave on the ECG is the T wave, which depicts ventricular repolarization (Figure 9.4). At times, a small complex known as the *U wave* may follow the T wave (see Figure 9.4). This is believed to represent the terminal stages of ventricular repolarization.

The segment between the QRS and the beginning of the T wave is known as the *ST segment*. The ST segment should be isoelectric, meaning it should be on the baseline and not show major upward

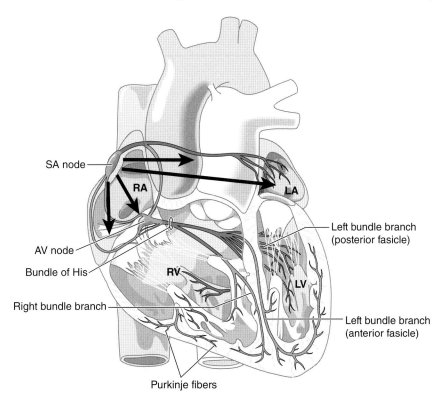

Figure 9.3 Electrical conduction system of the heart. Arrows indicate atrial depolarization. LA, left atrium; LV, left ventricle; RA, right atrium; RV, right ventricle; SA, sinoatrial. Source: Reprinted from Thompson WR, editor. *ACSM's Clinical Exercise Physiology*. Philadelphia (PA): Wolters Kluwer; 2018.

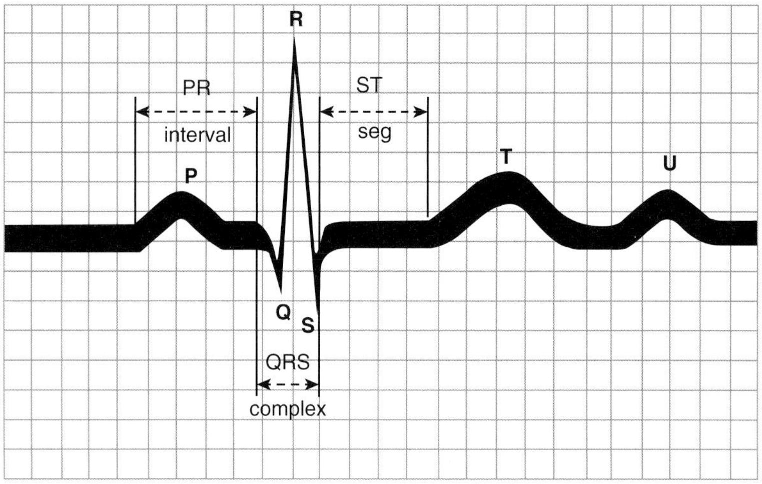

Figure 9.4 Waves, intervals, and segments of the normal ECG waveform. Source: Reprinted from Thompson WR, editor. *ACSM's Clinical Exercise Physiology*. Philadelphia (PA): Wolters Kluwer; 2018.

or downward deflections. ST-segment deviations have implications in the diagnosis of heart disease, depending on its deflection — elevation or depression.

The QT interval represents the return of stimulated ventricles to their resting state (ventricular repolarization). It is measured from the beginning of the QRS complex to the end of the T wave and is usually measured in the lead where it is the longest. The length of the QT interval will normally vary with heart rate (HR), so one normal value cannot be described. As the HR increases, the QT interval normally shortens; as the HR decreases, the QT interval lengthens. Therefore, the QT is typically measured as a function of the QT, or corrected for HR (QTc).

The corrected QT (QTc) interval takes into account the influence of the HR and tries to correct for it. Although several methods exist, the most widely used is the Bazett formula (3):

$$QTc = \frac{QT}{\sqrt{RR}}$$

where RR is the time between R-R intervals in seconds.

A simpler equation to calculate QTc has been proposed (4). Unlike the Bazett formula that requires a square root method, Hodges formula provides a linear relationship between QT and HR in milliseconds (Equation 1) or using seconds (Equation 2):

$$QTc\ (ms) = QT\ (ms) + 1.75\ (heart\ rate\ in\ beats\ per\ \min - 60) \qquad (1)$$

$$QTc\ (s) = QT\ (s) + 0.00175\ (heart\ rate\ in\ beats\ per\ \min - 60) \qquad (2)$$

Several other methods have been proposed to measure QTc (5). These methods seem to work best at HRs between 60 and 100 beats per minute (bpm). Nonetheless, caution is warranted when recording the QTc and trying to make clinical decisions, because these methods have shown to overcorrect at high HRs and undercorrect at low HRs (6,7).

Box 9.1	Normal Ranges for ECG Waveforms
P wave duration	≤120 ms (0.12 s)
P wave amplitude	≤0.25 mV (2.5 mm)
PR interval	120–200 ms (0.12–0.20 s)
QRS duration	<100 ms (0.10 s)
QTc	<450 ms (0.450 s)

Regardless of its potential inconsistencies, the measurement of QTc is an important surrogate for potential arrhythmias and should take into consideration when assessing ECG (6). Although the normal ranges may be debatable between men and women, a normal QTc is considered <0.45 seconds (<450 ms).

Although the details are beyond the scope of this chapter, it is important to note that the QT segment can be influenced by several factors (7), such as sex, with females having longer QT values than males (8); diurnal variations, where the QT is longest in the early morning (9); diet, where QT increases after a meal (10) and can be altered by consumption of protein supplements, caffeine, xanthine-containing products, chocolate, cocoa-containing drinks, alcoholic beverages, or grapefruit juice (11); certain pharmacological treatments; and electrolyte imbalances (*i.e.*, low potassium, magnesium, and calcium levels). Lastly, sympathetic and vagal activities that affect HR will impact the QT interval (12); thus, it is recommended individuals rest for 5 minutes in supine position before all ECG recording.

Lastly, the RR segment indicates the complete depolarization and repolarization of the myocardium and depicts a complete heart cycle. As a result, we can use the RR segment to more accurately calculate the HR.

Measuring Heart Rate

There are several methods to measure HR from the ECG. Here we discuss some of the most common.

Instantaneous Heart Rate Method

The instantaneous HR (IHR) method simply takes advantage of the time relationship between heart beats and provides a quick assessment of heart in a normal heart. To calculate IHR, divide the number of seconds in a minute (60) by the number of seconds between R-R intervals:

$$IHR\ (beats\ per\ min) = \frac{60}{RR\ (s)}$$

For example, if the distance between R-R intervals is 22 mm (22 small boxes), this is equal to 0.88 seconds (22 × 0.04 = 0.88 seconds). Therefore, 60/0.88 = 68 bpm. As long as the rate is consistent and one has a normal ECG, this method works well for a quick and relatively accurate measurement of HR.

1500 Method

A more accurate, but time-consuming, way to measure HR is the 1500 method. This technique allows the exercise physiologist the opportunity to accurately calculate HR when the rhythm is not constant and R-R variations exist. Using a 6- or 10-second ECG strip, one measures the distance (in millimeters) between multiple consecutive R-R intervals and then averages those values to calculate an HR (Figure 9.5).

At normal calibration (paper speed of 25 mm · s^{-1}), the distance between R-R intervals (in mm) divided into the constant 1500 yields the HR during that R-R interval (see Box 9.2 for an explanation of where the 1500-number comes from). For example, if the R-R interval is 22 mm, the HR during that interval is 68 bpm (1500/22 = 68.18).

If the R-R intervals are consistent, a single measurement between R-R can yield a good estimation of the average HR. However, if there is variation in the R-R intervals (this can be normal), R-R intervals should be measured and then averaged to determine a more accurate HR. For greatest accuracy, every R-R interval on the ECG strip should be measured and then averaged those calculated values to determine the average HR.

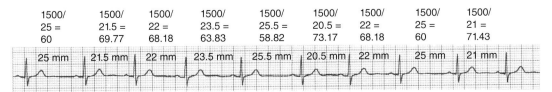

Figure 9.5 Calculating heart rate using the 1500 method. Source: Reprinted from Thompson WR, editor. *ACSM's Clinical Exercise Physiology*. Philadelphia (PA): Wolters Kluwer; 2018.

| Box 9.2 | Where Does the 1500-Number Come from? |

Remember, each small box is 1 mm in length and represents 0.04 seconds in time. Thus, if one were to run a 60-second ECG, there will be 1500 small boxes in that ECG. So, with this method, we can simply take a 10-second recording and calculate HR.

Box Counting Method

The box counting method is a simple way to calculate HR. In this method, one counts the number of large boxes between R-R intervals to determine the HR (Figure 9.6). This method is useful for a quick assessment of HR, as long as the R-R intervals appear in regular intervals. This is an important point because otherwise the estimation of HR will vary based on which R-R was chosen for the measurement.

To use this method, find the R wave that falls on a dark (thick) line — this will be your starting point. Then, find the next dark (thick) line. This is the 300 mark, and successive marks should be counted as 150-100-75-60-50-43-37-33. See Box 9.3 for a description of why these numbers are used.

Figure 9.7 provides an example of how to calculate HR using the box counting method. The reference R wave falls on a thick line near the starting of the ECG strip. After counting four dark (thick) lines, we encounter the next R wave, which is 1 mm passed the fourth dark (thick) line. If the second R wave would have fallen on the dark (thick) line, the HR would be estimated as 75 bpm. However, because the second R wave landed after the fourth dark (think) line, we know the estimated is between 75 and 60 bpm (between the fourth and fifth dark [thick] lines). Thus, we need to calculate the value of each thin line between the fourth and fifth dark (thick) lines. To do this, we take the difference between 75 and

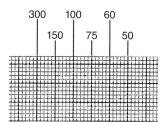

Figure 9.6 Calculating heart rate using the box method. Source: Reprinted from Thompson WR, editor. *ACSM's Clinical Exercise Physiology*. Philadelphia (PA): Wolters Kluwer; 2018.

| Box 9.3 | Where Does the Box Counting Method Come from? |

Remember the time periods of the ECG paper. One large box is equal to 0.20 seconds (0.04 seconds for each small box), and there are 5 small boxes in each large box (0.04 × 5 = 0.20 seconds). So, if we run a full 60-second ECG strip, there will be 300 large boxes. Therefore, the HR can be calculated based on the number of boxes between R-R waves as follows:

# Large Boxes	Time	ECG Interval
1	0.20 s/60 s	300
2	0.40 s/60 s	150
3	0.60 s/60 s	100
4	0.80 s/60 s	75
5	1.00 s/60 s	60
6	1.20 s/60 s	50
7	1.40 s/60 s	43
8	1.60 s/60 s	37.5
9	1.8 s/60 s	33

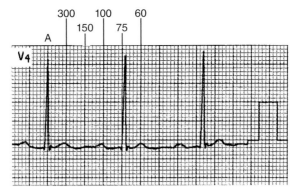

Figure 9.7 Example of heart rate estimation using the box method. Source: Reprinted from Thompson WR, editor. *ACSM's Clinical Exercise Physiology*. Philadelphia (PA): Wolters Kluwer; 2018.

60 (75 − 60 = 15) and divide this by the number of thin lines between the two thick (dark) lines, that is, 5. So, each thin line is a 3-bpm line (15/5); this suggests that the estimated HR for this individual is 72 bpm (75 − 3).

6-Second Method

For many individuals, a variable R-R interval is a normal rhythm. In this instance, many of the methods described earlier would not be accurate because they require little variability between R waves. Therefore, the 6-second method is most appropriate for variable rhythms. In this method, it is important to obtain a 6-second ECG strip to measure R waves. Today, this 6-second strip can be easily obtained, as ECG machines typically print 3-second marks at the bottom of the ECG paper (Figure 9.8).

To estimate HR, count the number of R-R intervals in 6 seconds, then multiply by 10. For example, in Figure 9.8, 6.5 R-R intervals are present in 6 seconds (note the vertical 3-second markers on the bottom of the strip); therefore, the HR is ~65 bpm. It is important to note that with this method, we are interested in counting the R-R intervals, not the R waves.

LEAD PLACEMENT AND PREPARATION FOR THE ELECTROCARDIOGRAM

The standard ECG consists of 12 views of the heart. Each view is established by a lead, in which each measure the same electrical events of myocardial depolarization and repolarization from different points of reference. The electrical events are the same, but viewed from different angles, which result in differing appearance for the respective ECG waves, such as the P waves, QRS complexes, T waves, and other events. Leads are discussed in detail later in this chapter.

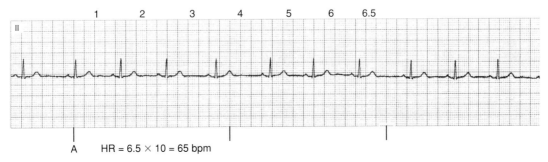

Figure 9.8 Six-second method of heart rate (HR) assessment. A represents 3-second marks in the ECG paper. Source: Adapted from Thompson WR, editor. *ACSM's Clinical Exercise Physiology*. Philadelphia (PA): Wolters Kluwer; 2018.

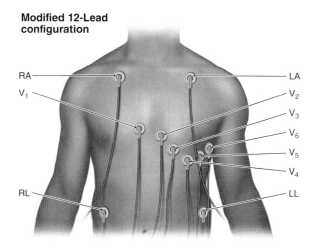

Figure 9.9 The Mason-Likar 12-lead ECG electrode placement for exercise testing. For females, the V4-V6 electrodes are typically placed on the chest wall underneath the lower portion of the breast. LA, left arm; LL, left leg; RA, right arm; RL, right leg.

The Leads

Even though several deviations from the standard ECG configuration exist, the Mason-Likar configuration is the most common for exercise testing (13). Several differences in interpretation exist between the standard and Mason-Likar configurations (14,15); however, those are also beyond the scope of this text.

To examine the ECG, 10 surface electrodes are placed on the chest, wrists, and ankles of a standard 12-lead ECG. To reduce noise from muscle contractions and for safety, the limb leads are modified and placed on the chest (the Mason-Likar lead system) during an exercise test. The wrist and ankle leads are replaced by leads in the subclavicular and suprailiac areas, respectively. See Figure 9.9 and Box 9.4 for details on lead placement of the Mason-Likar leads.

Each lead on an ECG records the electrical activity of the heart. Because the wave of depolarization has three-dimensional direction and a magnitude, the ECG signal measure is considered a vector. These vectors are influenced by several factors, such as the surface of the skin, muscle contractions, and

---

Box 9.4   Mason-Likar 12-Lead System

The Mason-Likar 10-electrode placement allows for conventional 12-lead exercise ECG tracings. The location of these electrodes is described as follows:

Right arm (RA): upper right arm-chest region immediately below the midpoint of the clavicle
Left arm (LA): upper left arm-chest region immediately below the midpoint of the clavicle
Right leg (RL): lower right abdominal region, at the midclavicular line, at the level of the last rib
Left leg (LL): lower left abdominal region, at the midclavicular line, at the level of the last rib
V1: fourth intercostal space at the right sternal border

Note: The fourth intercostal space can be found by locating the sternoclavicular joint and by placing the index finger in the space immediately below the first rib. This is the first intercostal space. Proceed down the sternum until the fourth space is found.

V2: fourth intercostal space at the left sternal border
V3: at the midpoint on a straight line between V2 and V4
V4: fifth intercostal space in the midclavicular line
V5: on the anterior axillary line, horizontal to V4
V6: on the midaxillary line, horizontal to both V4 and V5

The leg electrodes may also be placed at the level of the navel. However, there may be excessive motion artifact with this placement. Placement on the last rib at the midclavicular line tends to be more stable, with no effect on the ECG tracing.

Adapted from Kligfield P, Gettes LS, Bailey JJ, et al. Recommendations for the standardization and interpretation of the electrocardiogram: part I: the electrocardiogram and its technology a scientific statement from the American Heart Association Electrocardiography and Arrhythmias Committee, Council on Clinical Cardiology; the American College of Cardiology Foundation; and the Heart Rhythm Society Endorsed by the International Society for Computerized Electrocardiology. *J Am Coll Cardiol*. 2007;49(10):1109–27. doi:10.1016/j.jacc.2007.01.024.

movement. Thus, a resting ECG along with the individual resting quietly is paramount for accurate diagnosis. Moreover, it is also important to clean the area where each electrode will be placed with alcohol, and gentle abrasion before electrode application. This simple technique can help reduce noise and improve the quality of the recorded ECG (16).

The 12-lead ECG is made up of limb leads (I, II, III, aVR, aVL, and aVF) and chest leads (V1 through V6). It is worth noting that all leads are effectively "bipolar," and the term "unipolar" in reference to the chest leads lacks precision (16).

Limb Leads

Standard Limb Leads (I, II, III) The standard limb leads are made up of four electrodes placed on the wrist and ankles when using the standard ECG configuration, or below the clavicle and above the iliac crest when using the Mason-Likar configuration (Figure 9.9). The electrode placed on the right ankle is considered a ground electrode and does not provide any electrical conduction. Each lead records voltage between the two extremities and collectively create a triangle, commonly known as Einthoven triangle, after William Einthoven (1860–1927), a Dutch physiologist and physicist who invented ECG (17).

Lead I connects the right arm (RA) and left arm (LA), Lead II connects the RA to the left leg (LL), and Lead III connects the LA with the LL (Figure 9.10). Each lead records the difference in voltage between electrodes, and the ECG amplifies this signal into the ECG paper. Considering the relationship of all the three leads, the voltage of any wave in Lead I added to the voltage in Lead III equals the voltage in Lead II (LI + LIII = LII). One can simply test this equation by looking at the voltage of the R wave in Lead I and the voltage of the R wave in Lead III and you should get the voltage of the R wave in Lead II. (Note: This can also be done with the voltages of the P waves and T waves.)

Augmented limb leads (aVR, aVL, and aVF) The augmented leads are an extension of the standard limb leads. Although these leads are often considered unipolar, they are bipolar in nature, as they simply record the electrical voltages at one location relative to an electrode with close to zero potential. In other words, when the three augmented limb leads are recorded, their voltages should total zero (aVR + aVL + aVF = 0). Because the sum of the voltages of RA, LA, and LL equals zero, the central terminal has a zero voltage (18). These leads are considered "augmented" because the electrocardiograph augments 50% of the actual voltages at each extremity.

Each augmented lead measures voltage deviations from a positive electrode — RA for aVR, LA for aVL, and LL for aVF — to a negative electrode composed of the combination of the other two electrodes in the system (Figure 9.10).

Chest Leads (V1-V6)

The chest leads, also known as *pericardial or ventral leads*, are placed on the chest and record the electrical activity toward the positive electrodes on the chest, from an imaginary "negative" pole in the center of the heart.

Each lead records electrical activity from a specific area of the heart. For example, V1 records electrical activity from the right side of the septum, V2 records from the anterior side of the heart and septum, V3 and V4 record from the anterior region of the heart, whereas V5 and V6 record electrical activity from the lateral region of the heart (Figure 9.10).

The ECG provides an electrical view of the heart in the transverse (horizontal), frontal (vertical), and sagittal (lateral) planes. Figure 9.10 shows a normal ECG complex with associated representation of the anatomic correlates for each wave. A view of the heart in the vertical plane is derived from information received from the limb electrodes, which produce the six limb leads (I, II, III, aVR, aVL, and aVF). The six chest leads (V1–V6) show the heart in a horizontal plane. Leads II, III, and aVF view the inferior surface of the heart; leads V1–V4 view the anterior surface of the heart; and leads I, aVL, V5, and V6 view the lateral surface of the heart. By examining the ECG in more than one plane and lead, normal and abnormal function of the myocardium can be determined (Figure 9.11).

Artifacts from movement, electrical interference, and poor skin preparation can significantly affect the quality of both resting and exercise ECG. It is extremely important to minimize all artifacts through proper skin preparation, precise electrode placement, and standardized operating conditions within ECG and exercise testing facilities.

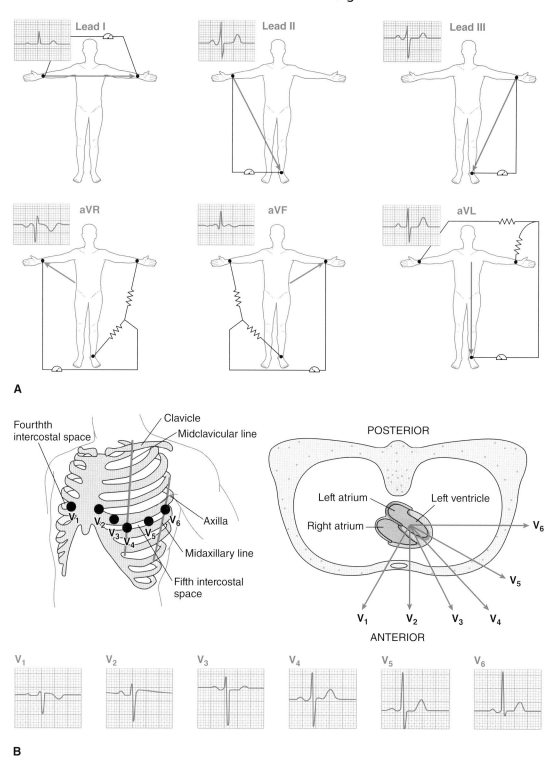

Figure 9.10 The standard ECG and its view of the heart. **A:** Frontal plane leads. **B:** Transverse plane-precordial leads. Source: Reprinted from Boron WF, Boulpaep EL, editors. *Medical Physiology,* 3rd ed. Philadelphia (PA): Elsevier; 2016. Figure 21.8.

CARDIAC RHYTHMS

As mentioned previously, the context in this chapter provides an exploratory look at the ECG and should be used as an introduction in the topic. As such, we provide a detailed overview of the basic concepts to get students started. The following sections provide insight to what constitutes a sinus (normal) ECG rhythm and some rate variations.

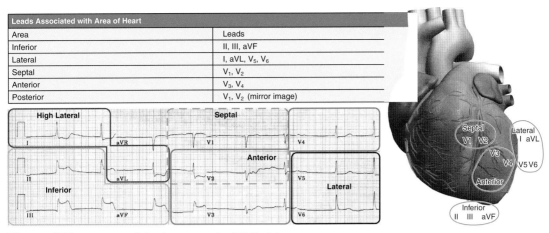

Leads Associated with Area of Heart	
Area	Leads
Inferior	II, III, aVF
Lateral	I, aVL, V$_5$, V$_6$
Septal	V$_1$, V$_2$
Anterior	V$_3$, V$_4$
Posterior	V$_1$, V$_2$ (mirror image)

Figure 9.11 Regions of the heart on the ECG strip.

Sinus Rhythm

"Normal sinus rhythm" is indicative of a normal rhythm originating at the SA node. Therefore, the ECG waves all appear in order (P wave, QRS complex, T wave), with a rate between 60 and 100 bpm. Rates slower than 60 bpm are referred to as *bradycardia*, and those faster than 100 bpm are termed *tachycardia*. Both rhythms are considered to be "normal" depending on the individual and the situation. For example, sinus tachycardia with rates around 150 to 200 bpm may be entirely normal in the context of exercise, yet abnormal for an individual with coronary artery disease (CAD) at rest. Likewise, bradycardia with rates lower than 50 bpm — and even less than 40 bpm in some cases — may occur asymptomatically and without problem in highly trained endurance athletes; however, in an individual with significant myocardial pathology, brady-cardia may indicate β-blockade therapy, the presence of a rhythm disturbance, or other clinical condition.

Bradycardias

Sinus bradycardia occurs when the impulse originates from the sinus node at a rate <60 bpm. This may be present in trained individuals with high parasympathetic (vagal) tone, in patients who are receiving drugs that slow the HR (*e.g.*, β-blockers), or in individuals who have disease of the sinus node (*e.g.*, sick sinus syndrome). Most bradycardias are related to physiologic or neurogenic factors, including increased vagal tone related to physical fitness (*e.g.*, the slow-resting HR of many endurance athletes) or other mechanisms that affect parasympathetic/sympathetic tone. This type of bradycardia is rarely clinically significant in the absence of heart disease or other myocardial pathology.

Sinus Tachycardia

Sinus tachycardia is defined by a rate >100 bpm and is the result of an enhanced firing rate of the sinus node. Sinus tachycardia results when increased activity of the sympathetic nervous system is present, including during times of fear, exercise, fever, hypovolemia, bleeding, hypoxia, or other acute illness. Decreased stroke volume related to severe left ventricular dysfunction may also result in sinus tachy-cardia due to sympathetic nervous system activation in an attempt to preserve adequate cardiac output. Three key features of sinus tachycardia are important. First, patients typically exhibit a gradual increase in HR (*e.g.*, sudden acceleration from 80 to 150 bpm does not occur). Second, although exceptions occur, the sinus rate typically does not exceed the maximum HR. Third, the P wave must be normal.

SUMMARY

In this chapter, we have attempted to provide an introduction to basic and fundamental methods of electrocardiography. We acknowledge there are many important concepts not included here; however, we believe those are beyond the scope of this text. This chapter should serve as an introduction to ECGs and its potential role in identifying abnormal ECG rhythms. For a more detailed description of ECG concepts, the reader is referred to the work of Dunbar and colleagues (1,2).

LABORATORY ACTIVITIES

Electrocardiography

Activity 1: Using the diagram provided, identify the location of the 10 electrodes that constitute the 12 leads of the ECG. Mark each location with an "X" (19).

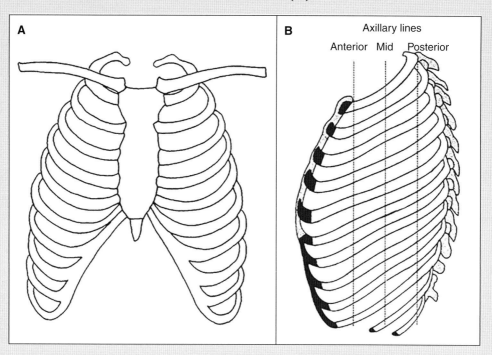

Using the ECGs provided, practice reading ECGs and answer the following questions.

ECG 1:

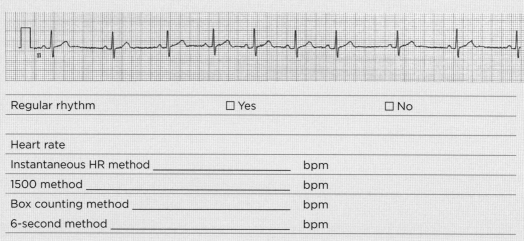

Regular rhythm	☐ Yes	☐ No

Heart rate

Instantaneous HR method _____ bpm

1500 method _____ bpm

Box counting method _____ bpm

6-second method _____ bpm

| Rhythm description | ☐ Normal (sinus) | ☐ Bradycardia | ☐ Tachycardia |

| P wave | Duration _____ mm | Amplitude _____ mm |

| PR interval measures _____ mm | _____ s |

| QRS complex measures _____ mm | _____ s |

| Q waves | ☐ Yes | ☐ No |

| QTc interval | _____ s | _____ ms |

| ST segment | ☐ Isoelectric | ☐ Elevation | ☐ Depression |

Credit: Dr. Trisha VanDusseldorp, Kennesaw State University

ECG 2:

| Regular rhythm | ☐ Yes | ☐ No |

Heart rate

| Instantaneous HR method _____ bpm |
| 1500 method _____ bpm |
| Box counting method _____ bpm |
| 6-second method _____ bpm |

| Rhythm description | ☐ Normal (sinus) | ☐ Bradycardia | ☐ Tachycardia |

| P wave | Duration _____ mm | Amplitude _____ mm |

| PR interval measures _____ mm | _____ s |

| QRS complex measures _____ mm | _____ s |

| Q waves | ☐ Yes | ☐ No |

| QTc interval | _____ s | _____ ms |

| ST segment | ☐ Isoelectric | ☐ Elevation | ☐ Depression |

Credit: Dr. Trisha VanDusseldorp, Kennesaw State University

(*continued*)

LABORATORY ACTIVITIES (*continued*)

ECG 3:

Regular rhythm	☐ Yes	☐ No

Heart rate

Instantaneous HR method _____ bpm

1500 method _____ bpm

Box counting method _____ bpm

6-second method _____ bpm

Rhythm description	☐ Normal (sinus)	☐ Bradycardia	☐ Tachycardia

P wave   Duration _____ mm   Amplitude _____ mm

PR interval measures _____ mm   _____ s

QRS complex measures _____ mm   _____ s

Q waves	☐ Yes	☐ No

QTc interval   _____ s   _____ ms

ST segment	☐ Isoelectric	☐ Elevation ☐ Depression

Credit: Dr. Trisha VanDusseldorp, Kennesaw State University

ECG 4:

Regular rhythm	☐ Yes	☐ No

Heart rate

Instantaneous HR method _____ bpm

1500 method _____ bpm

Box counting method _____ bpm

6-second method _____ bpm

Rhythm description	☐ Normal (Sinus)	☐ Bradycardia	☐ Tachycardia

P wave	Duration _____ mm	Amplitude _____ mm

PR interval measures _____ mm		_____ s

QRS complex measures _____ mm		_____ s

Q waves	☐ Yes	☐ No

QTc interval	_____ s	_____ ms

ST segment	☐ Isoelectric	☐ Elevation ☐ Depression

Credit: Dr. Trisha VanDusseldorp, Kennesaw State University

ECG 5:

Regular rhythm	☐ Yes	☐ No

Heart rate

Instantaneous HR method _____ bpm
1500 method _____ bpm
Box counting method _____ bpm
6-second method _____ bpm

Rhythm description ☐ Normal (sinus)	☐ Bradycardia	☐ Tachycardia

P wave	Duration _____ mm	Amplitude _____ mm

PR interval measures _____ mm		_____ s

QRS complex measures _____ mm		_____ s

Q waves	☐ Yes	☐ No

QTc interval	_____ s	_____ ms

ST segment	☐ Isoelectric	☐ Elevation	☐ Depression

Credit: Dr. Trisha VanDusseldorp, Kennesaw State University

REFERENCES

1. Dunbar CC. Electrocardiography. In: Thompson WR, editor. *ACSM's Clinical Exercise Physiology*. Philadelphia (PA): Wolters Kluwer; 2019. p. 205–89.
2. Dunbar C, Saul B. *ECG Interpretation for the Clinical Exercise Physiologist*. Philadelphia (PA): Wolters Kluwer; 2009.
3. Bazett H. An analysis of the time-relations of electrocardiograms. *Ann Noninvasive Electrocardiol*. 1997;2(2):177–94.
4. Hodges M. Rate correction of the QT interval. *Card Electrophysiol Rev*. 1997;1(3):360–3. doi:10.1023/A:1009933509868.
5. Postema PG, Wilde AA. The measurement of the QT interval. *Curr Cardiol Rev*. 2014;10(3):287–94. doi:10.2174/1573403x10666140514103612.
6. Malik M. Problems of heart rate correction in assessment of drug-induced QT interval prolongation. *J Cardiovasc Electrophysiol*. 2001;12(4):411–20. doi:10.1046/j.1540-8167.2001.00411.x.
7. Salvi V, Karnad DR, Panicker GK, Kothari S. Update on the evaluation of a new drug for effects on cardiac repolarization in humans: issues in early drug development. *Br J Pharmacol*. 2010;159(1):34–48. doi:10.1111/j.1476-5381.2009.00427.x.
8. Stramba-Badiale M, Locati E, Martinelli A, Courville J, Schwartz P. Gender and the relationship between ventricular repolarization and cardiac cycle length during 24-h Holter recordings. *Eur Heart J*. 1997;18(6):1000–6.
9. Molnar J, Zhang F, Weiss J, Ehlert FA, Rosenthal JE. Diurnal pattern of QTc interval: how long is prolonged? Possible relation to circadian triggers of cardiovascular events. *J Am Coll Cardiol*. 1996;27(1):76–83.
10. Nagy D, DeMeersman R, Gallagher D, et al. QTc interval (cardiac repolarization): lengthening after meals. *Obes Res*. 1997;5(6):531–7. doi:10.1002/j.1550-8528.1997.tb00573.x.
11. Zitron E, Scholz E, Owen RW, et al. QTc prolongation by grapefruit juice and its potential pharmacological basis: HERG channel blockade by flavonoids. *Circulation*. 2005;111(7):835–8.
12. Magnano AR, Holleran S, Ramakrishnan R, Reiffel JA, Bloomfield DM. Autonomic nervous system influences on QT interval in normal subjects. *J Am Coll Cardiol*. 2002;39(11):1820–6. doi:10.1016/s0735-1097(02)01852-1.
13. Papouchado M, Walker P, James M, Clarke L. Fundamental differences between the standard 12-lead electrocardiograph and the modified (Mason-Likar) exercise lead system. *Eur Heart J*. 1987;8(7):725–33.
14. Sevilla DC, Dohrmann ML, Somelofski CA, Wawrzynski RP, Wagner NB, Wagner GS. Invalidation of the resting electrocardiogram obtained via exercise electrode sites as a standard 12-lead recording. *Am J Cardiol*. 1989;63(1):35–9.
15. Welinder A, Sörnmo L, Feild DQ, et al. Comparison of signal quality between Easi and Mason-Likar 12-lead electrocardiograms during physical activity. *Am J Crit Care*. 2004;13(3):228–34. doi:10.4037/ajcc2004.13.3.228.
16. Kligfield P, Gettes LS, Bailey JJ, et al. Recommendations for the standardization and interpretation of the electrocardiogram: part I: the electrocardiogram and its technology a scientific statement from the American Heart Association Electrocardiography and Arrhythmias Committee, Council on Clinical Cardiology; the American College of Cardiology Foundation; and the Heart Rhythm Society Endorsed by the International Society for Computerized Electrocardiology. *J Am Coll Cardiol*. 2007;49(10):1109–27. doi:10.1016/j.jacc.2007.01.024.
17. Barold SS. Willem Einthoven and the birth of clinical electrocardiography a hundred years ago. *Card Electrophysiol Rev*. 2003;7(1):99–104. doi:10.1023/a:1023667812925.
18. Goldberger AL, Goldberger ZD, Shvilkin A. ECG leads. In: Goldberger AL, Goldberger ZD, Shvilkin A, editors. *Goldberger's Clinical Electrocardiography: A Simplified Approach*. Philadelphia, PA: Elsevier; 2018.
19. Rajaganeshan R, Ludlam CL, Francis DP, Parasramka SV, Sutton R. Accuracy in ECG lead placement among technicians, nurses, general physicians and cardiologists. *Int J Clin Prac*. 2007;62(1):65–70. doi:10.1111/j.1742-1241.2007.01390..x.

A Conversions

LENGTH OR HEIGHT

1 kilometer = 1000 meters (m)
1 kilometer = 0.62137 miles
1 mile = 1609.35 meters
1 meter = 100 centimeters (cm) = 1000 millimeters (mm)
1 foot = 0.3048 meters
1 meter = 3.281 feet = 39.37 inches
1 inch = 2.54 centimeters
0.394 inches = 1 centimeter

MASS OR WEIGHT

1 kilogram = 1000 grams (g) = 10 Newtons (N)
1 kilogram = 2.2 pounds
1 pound = 0.454 kilograms
1 gram = 1000 milligrams (mg)
1 pound = 453.592 grams
1 ounce = 28.3495 grams
1 gram = 0.035 ounces

VOLUME

1 liter = 1000 milliliters (mL)
1 liter = 1.05 quarts
1 quart = 0.9464 liters
1 milliliter = 1 cubic centimeter (cc or cm^3)
1 gallon = 3.785 liters (L)

WORK

1 Newton-meter = 1 Joule (J)
1 Newton-meter = 0.7375 foot-pounds
1 foot-pound = 1.36 Newton-meters
1 kilojoule (1000 J) = 0.234 kilocalories (kcal)
1 foot-pound = 0.1383 kilograms per meter ($kg \cdot m^{-1}$)
1 $kg \cdot m^{-1}$ = 7.23 foot-pounds

VELOCITY

1 meter per second ($m \cdot s^{-1}$) = 2.2372 miles per hour ($mi \cdot h^{-1}$)
1 mile per hour = 26.8 meters per minute ($m \cdot min^{-1}$) = 1.6093 kilometers per hour ($km \cdot h^{-1}$)

POWER

1 kilogram-meter per minute ($kg \cdot m^{-1} \cdot min^{-1}$) = 0.1635 watts (W)

1 watt = 6.12 $kg \cdot m^{-1} \cdot min^{-1}$

1 $kg \cdot m^{-1} \cdot min^{-1}$ = 1 $kp \cdot m^{-1} \cdot min^{-1}$

1 watt = 1 Joule per second ($J \cdot s^{-1}$)

1 horsepower (hp) = 745.7 watts

TEMPERATURE

1° C = 1° Kelvin (K) = 1.8° F

1° F = 0.56° C

METRIC ROOTS

deci = 1/10

centi = 1/100

milli = 1/1000

kilo = 1000

---

[1] The Preparticipation Screening Algorithm and Exercise Preparticipation Health Screening Questionnaire for Exercise Professionals are used with permission from ACSM. All other forms are used with the permission of the Ball State University Clinical Exercise Physiology Program.

PREPARTICIPATION SCREENING ALGORITHM

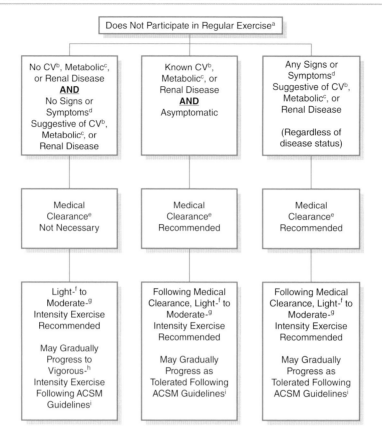

^aExercise Participation   Performing planned, structured physical activity for at least 30 min at moderate intensity on at least 3 d · wk⁻¹ for at least the last 3 mo

ᵃExercise Participation — Performing planned, structured physical activity for at least 30 min at moderate intensity on at least 3 d · wk⁻¹ for at least the last 3 mo

ᵇCV Disease — Cardiac, peripheral vascular, or cerebrovascular disease

ᶜMetabolic Disease — Type 1 and Type 2 diabetes mellitus

ᵈSigns and Symptoms — At rest or during activity. Includes pain, discomfort in the chest, neck, jaw, arms, or other areas that may result from ischemia; shortness of breath at rest or with mild exertion; dizziness or syncope; orthopnea or paroxysmal nocturnal dyspnea; ankle edema; palpitations or tachycardia; intermittent claudication; known heart murmur; unusual fatigue or shortness of breath with usual activities.

ᵉMedical Clearance — Approval from a health care professional to engage in exercise.

ᶠLight-Intensity Exercise — 30%–39% HRR or $\dot{V}O_2R$, 2–2.9 METs, RPE 9–11, an intensity that causes slight increases in HR and breathing

ᵍModerate-Intensity Exercise — 40%–59% HRR or $\dot{V}O_2R$, 3–5.9 METs, RPE 12–13, an intensity that causes noticeable increases in HR and breathing

ʰVigorous-Intensity Exercise — 60% HRR or $\dot{V}O_2R$, ≥6 METs, RPE ≥14, an intensity that causes substantial increases in HR and breathing

ⁱACSM Guidelines — See the most current edition of *ACSM's Guidelines for Exercise Testing and Prescription*

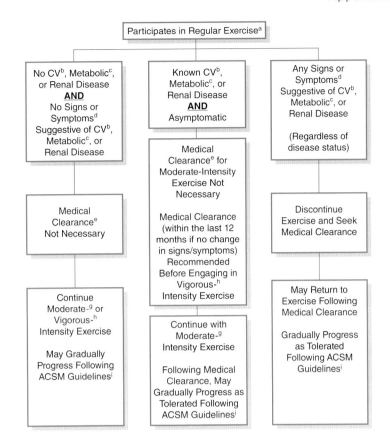

^aExercise Participation   Performing planned, structured physical activity for at least 30 min at moderate
                                          intensity on at least 3 d · wk⁻¹ for at least the last 3 mo
^bCV Disease   Cardiac, peripheral vascular, or cerebrovascular disease
^cMetabolic Disease   Type 1 and Type 2 diabetes mellitus
^dSigns and Symptoms   At rest or during activity. Includes pain, discomfort in the chest, neck, jaw, arms,
                                          or other areas that may result from ischemia; shortness of breath at rest or with
                                          mild exertion; dizziness or syncope; orthopnea or paroxysmal nocturnal
                                          dyspnea; ankle edema; palpitations or tachycardia; intermittent claudication;
                                          known heart murmur; unusual fatigue or shortness of breath with usual activities.
^eMedical Clearance   Approval from a health care professional to engage in exercise.
^fLight-Intensity Exercise   30%–39% HRR or V̇O₂R, 2–2.9 METs, RPE 9–11, an intensity that causes slight
                                          increases in HR and breathing
^gModerate-Intensity Exercise 40%–59% HRR or V̇O₂R, 3–5.9 METs, RPE 12–13, an intensity that causes
                                          noticeable increases in HR and breathing
^hVigorous-Intensity Exercise 60% HRR or V̇O₂R, ≥6 METs, RPE ≥14, an intensity that causes substantial
                                          increases in HR and breathing
ⁱACSM Guidelines   See the most current edition of *ACSM's Guidelines for Exercise Testing and Prescription*

EXERCISE PREPARTICIPATION HEALTH SCREENING QUESTIONNAIRE FOR EXERCISE PROFESSIONALS

Assess your client's health needs by marking all *true* statements.
Step 1

SIGNS AND SYMPTOMS
Does your client experience:

____ chest discomfort with exertion

____ unreasonable breathlessness

____ dizziness, fainting, blackouts

____ ankle swelling

____ unpleasant awareness of a forceful, rapid, or irregular heart rate

____ burning or cramping sensations in their lower legs when walking short distance

____ known heart murmur

If you **did** mark any of these statements under the symptoms, **STOP**, your client should seek medical clearance before engaging in or resuming exercise. Your client may need to use a facility with a **medically qualified staff**.

If you did not mark any symptoms, move on to Steps 2 and 3.

Step 2

CURRENT ACTIVITY
Has your client performed planned, structured physical activity for at least 30 min at moderate intensity on at least 3 d wk^{-1} for at least 3 mo ?
Yes ☐   No ☐
Move on to Step 3.

Step 3

MEDICAL CONDITIONS
Has your client had or do they currently have:

__a heart attack

__heart surgery, cardiac catheterization, or coronary angioplasty

__pacemaker/implantable cardiac defibrillator/rhythm disturbance

__heart valve disease

__heart failure

__heart transplantation

__congenital heart disease

__diabetes

__renal disease

Evaluating Steps 2 and 3:

- If you **did not mark any of the statements in Step 3**, medical clearance is not necessary.
- If you marked Step 2 "**yes**" and **marked any of the statements in Step 3**, your client may continue to exercise at light-to-moderate intensity without medical clearance. Medical clearance is recommended before engaging in vigorous exercise.
- If you marked Step 2 "**no**" and **marked any of the statements in Step 3**, medical clearance is recommended. Your client may need to use a facility with a **medically qualified staff**.

BODY COMPOSITION DATA FORM

Client Name	Date	Technician(s)	File #

Weight History Review	**Visual Impression Record**

Weight at age 18 _____ lbs

   Cyclic Wt Loss? Y/N

Recent Wt Loss? Y/N if yes (lbs, time) _____

Previous Body Comp. Data (% fat, wt, date) _____

% fat appearance: (circle one)

   <10 10–15 15–20 20–25 25–30 >30

Overall appearance:

   Lean / Muscular / Average / Fat

Body Comp Considerations

   Exercise (last 3 hrs): Y/N   Eating (last 3 hrs): Y/N   Void (last 1 hr): Y/N

Height/Weight

Weight (nearest 0.25 lb) ____ lb   /   2.2046 = ____ kg

Height (nearest 0.25 in) ____ in   ×   0.0254 = ____ m

Body Mass Index (kg · m^{-2}) ____ kg / (____ m × ____ m) = ____

Circumference (cm)

	1	2	3	Mean	
Waist	____	____	____	____	Waist-to-Hip Ratio: _____
Hip	____	____	____	____	

Skinfold (mm)

Sex	Site	1	2	3	Mean	
W	Triceps	____	____	____	____	**Body Density: 1.__ __ __**
W	Suprailiac	____	____	____	____	
W	Thigh	____	____	____	____	***%Fat (3 site):** _____
	alternate	____	____	____	____	
M	Chest	____	____	____	____	Staff Comments:_____
M	Abdomen	____	____	____	____	_____
M	Thigh	____	____	____	____	_____

*See below: *Three-Site Formula* and *Conversion of Body Density (Db) to Percent Body Fat*

Three-Site Skinfold Formulas by gender:

Men: Body Density = 1.112 − 0.00043499 (SSF__) + 0.00000055 (SSF__)² − 0.00028826 (Age__)

Women: Body Density = 1.097 − 0.00046971 (SSF__) + 0.00000056 (SSF__)² − 0.00012828
         (Age__)

Body Density (Db) to Percent Body Fat Conversion by age/gender:

Men ages 20–80 yrs: (4.95/Db) − 4.50

Women ages 20–80 yrs: (5.01/Db) − 4.57

Staff Comments: _____

MUSCULAR FITNESS DATA FORM

_____   _____   _____   _____
Client Name   Date   Technician(s)   File #

Age: _____   Gender: _____   Weight: _____ lb _____ kg   Height: _____ in _____ cm

Strength Assessment

Right Hand Grip Strength

Trial 1 (kg)	Trial 2 (kg)	Trial 3 (kg)	**Best Score (kg)**
_____	_____	_____	_____

Left Hand Grip Strength

Trial 1 (kg)	Trial 2 (kg)	Trial 3 (kg)	**Best Score (kg)**
_____	_____	_____	_____

Combined Score: _____   Classification: _____

1-RM Bench Press Strength

Trial 1 (kg)	Trial 2 (kg)	Trial 3 (kg)	**Best Score (kg)**	**Ratio**
_____	_____	_____	_____	_____

Classification: _____

1-RM Leg Press Strength

Trial 1 (kg)	Trial 2 (kg)	Trial 3 (kg)	**Best Score (kg)**	**Ratio**
_____	_____	_____	_____	_____

Classification: _____

Endurance Assessment

Submaximal Bench Press

Total Number of Lifts _____

Classification: _____

Push-Up Test

Total Number of Push-Ups _____

Classification: _____

FLEXIBILITY DATA FORM

_____ _____ _____ _____
Client Name   Date   Technician(s)   File #

Age: _____ Gender: _____ Weight: _____ lb _____ kg Height: _____ in _____ cm

Trial 1 (in)   Trial 2 (in)   Trial 3 (in)   **Best Score (in)**
_____   _____   _____   _____

"Zero" Point: _____ Inches   Classification: _____

Trial 1 (cm)   Trial 2 (cm)   Trial 3 (cm)   **Best Score (cm)**
_____   _____   _____   _____

"Zero" Point: _____ cm   Classification: _____

| Lumbar Extension Test |

Trial 1 (in)   Trial 2 (in)   Trial 3 (in)   **Best Score (in)**
_____   _____   _____   _____

Classification: _____

| Lumbar Flexion Test |

Trial 1 (in)   Trial 2 (in)   Trial 3 (in)   **Best Score (in)**
_____   _____   _____   _____

Classification: _____

Range of Motion Assessments

Flexibility Test	Measured Range of Motion
Shoulder Flexion	
Shoulder Extension	
Shoulder Internal Rotation	
Shoulder External Rotation	
Hip Flexion (testing leg fully extended)	
Hip Flexion (testing knee flexed 90^0 and hip flexed 90^0)	
Hip Extension (testing leg fully extended)	
Hip Abduction	
Hip Adduction	

SUBMAXIMAL CYCLE TEST DATA FORM

Name: _____ Age: _____ Sex: _____ Date: _____

Time of test: _____ ID #: _____

Rest HR: _____ Rest BP: _____

supine / sitting*   supine / sitting*

Weight: _____ lb _____ kg   Height: _____ in _____ cm

Hours since last meal _____ List food and/or beverages: _____

MEDICATIONS: Dose   Time last taken

_____

_____

_____

ACTIVITY/EXERCISE HISTORY: _____

PAST ET: Date: _____ HR_{max}: _____ BP_{max}: _____/_____ $\dot{V}O_{2max}$: _____ Test Time: _____ Protocol: _____

Minute	Resistance (kg)	kg·m·min⁻¹	Pulse Palpation (15 s)	HR Monitor (bpm)	BP (mm Hg)	RPE
1						
2						
3						
4						
5						
6						
7						
8						
9						
10						
11						
12						
Recovery 1						
Recovery 2						
Recovery 3						

Estimated $\dot{V}O_{2max}$: _____

Fitness Classification: _____

*Use standing for a treadmill test.

EXERCISE TEST DATA FORM

Name: _____ Age: _____ Sex: _____ Date: _____

Time of test: _____ ID #: _____

Rest HR: _____ Rest BP: _____

              supine / sitting*   supine / sitting*

Weight: _____ lb _____ kg   Height: _____ in _____ cm

Hours since last meal _____   List food and/or beverages: _____

MEDICATIONS: Dose   Time last taken

_____
_____
_____

ACTIVITY/EXERCISE HISTORY: _____

PAST ET: Date: _____ HR_{max}: _____ BP_{max}: _____/_____ $\dot{V}O_{2max}$: _____ Test Time: _____ Protocol: _____

Protocol: _____

Time (min)	Work Setting	HR (bmp)	BP (mmHg)	RPE	Comments
0–1	/		/		
1–2	/		/		
2–3	/		/		
3–4	/		/		
4–5	/		/		
5–6	/		/		
6–7	/		/		
7–8	/		/		
8–9	/		/		
10–11	/		/		
11–12	/		/		
13–14	/		/		
Immediate Posttest Symptoms: Chest Discomfort		**SOB**		**Light-headedness**	**Other**
Recovery				**ACTIVE or SUPINE**	
0–1			/		
1–2			/		
2–3			/		
3–4			/		
4–5			/		

REASON for STOPPING TEST: _____

TECH 1:_____ TECH 2: _____ SUPERVISOR: _____

Note: work setting is speed and grade for the treadmill or resistance and rpm for the cycle.
*Use standing for a treadmill test.

PREPARTICIPATION HEALTH SCREENING AND EVALUATION

- Todd is a 44-year-old, married, electrical engineer who works 50 to 60 h · wk^{-1}. He is 5 ft. 9 in and weighs 233 lb, with total cholesterol of 192 mg · dL^{-1}, low-density lipoprotein (LDL) of 138 mg · dL^{-1}, HDL of 41 mg · dL^{-1}, triglycerides of 200 mg · dL^{-1}, and blood glucose of 120 mg · dL^{-1}. Todd's resting heart rate (HR) is 81 beats per minute (bpm) and blood pressure is 144/86 mm Hg. His waist and hip circumference measures are 42 and 40 in, respectively. Todd has never smoked but usually has one to two glasses of wine with dinner. He reports no leisure-time physical activity and does not exercise on a regular basis (less than two sessions per month). Todd denies all complaints of chest discomfort and shortness of breath at rest or with exertion; however, he has gained 20 lb over the past 2 years. Todd also has obstructive sleep apnea and is being treated with continuous positive airway pressure. A review of his family history reveals that Todd's father had a double bypass surgery at the age of 53 years and had a fatal myocardial infarction at the age of 62 years. Todd's brother (42-year-old) is hypertensive and was recently diagnosed with Type 2 diabetes, which is being treated with diet and physical activity recommendations. Todd has been referred to your facility for coronary artery disease risk factor reduction and physical activity counseling.
  - Determine the presence or absence of each cardiovascular disease (CVD) risk factor, any signs or symptoms suggestive of disease, and the recommendation for medical clearance before a fitness assessment or initiating exercise.
- Jerome, a 29-year-old college graduate, participated in a health screening at his local fitness center, where they performed a finger stick to evaluate cholesterol and blood glucose. Jerome's results reported that his total cholesterol was 287 mg · dL^{-1} and his HDL was 43 mg · dL^{-1}. It turns out that Jerome was not aware of the need to fast before the finger stick, nor did the test provide a value for LDL cholesterol. Given Jerome's high cholesterol values, it was advised to repeat the test on a different day, after a period of fasting, which, in fact, he did arrange for. His follow-up results were total cholesterol, 265 mg · dL^{-1}; HDL, 38 mg · dL^{-1}; triglycerides, 185 mg · dL^{-1}; LDL, 190 mg · dL^{-1}, and glucose, 106 mg · dL^{-1}.
  - Provide an interpretation of these tests and explain what recommendation you would make to Jerome.
- Jerome was a baseball player at a small college and has tried to maintain his college fitness over the past few years. When he went for his follow-up blood test, he also received a printout of body mass index (BMI), which was calculated based on his height of 5ft. 11 in. and his weight of 188 lb, and determined to be "overweight."
  - Calculate Jerome's BMI.
  - Knowing Jerome's BMI and assuming his waist circumference is 96 cm, what would you suggest to him based on this information?

BODY COMPOSITION

- David and Janessa came to the ABC Fitness Center to have their body composition measured via underwater weighing. However, they first need to have their respective residual volumes measured, based on the following:
  - David: age — 35 years, gender — male, height 71 in
  - Janessa: age — 36 years, gender — female, height 66 in

  In addition, because the density of the water varies with temperature, the temperature of the water needs to be measured. The density of water at a specific temperature can then be determined using various Web site calculators.

  Typically, a freestanding tank of water and mechanical scale are used for the underwater weighing procedure. Load cell scales can also be used for hydrostatic weighing, but are not as common. The mechanical scale is attached to a chair that sits inside the water tank for seating the client. The scale remains outside the water at all times while the client is weighed (see Figure 3.4). The assessment procedures for underwater weighing are provided in Box 3.1. Owing to the effort required to maximally exhale while being submerged underwater, the results of this test are dependent on the client's effort and success in performing the technique correctly; therefore, a margin of error does exist. The formula for calculating body volume from this procedure is as follows:

$$\text{Body volume} = \left\{ \frac{\left[\text{Body weight (g)} - \text{Underweight (g)}\right]}{\text{Water density (g / cm}^3)} \right\} - [\text{Residual volume (mL)} + 100 \text{ mL}]$$

Finally, body weight is divided by body volume to derive body density (Db).

- Given that David weighs 187 lb with a body volume of 81.5 L, and Janessa weighs 142 lb with a body volume of 62.2 L, calculate the Db for each.
- Using the appropriate equation in Table 3.1, calculate the body fat percent for David, who is African American, and also for Janessa, who is Hispanic.
- Shaun and Amanda also came to the ABC Fitness Center to have their body fat measured and have asked to have their skinfolds measured to determine body fat. Using the information in Box 3.3, calculate the body fat of Shaun (male, 28-year-old) and Amanda (female, 31-year-old) based on the following:
  - Shaun: chest — 11 cm, abdomen — 28 cm, thigh — 19 cm
  - Amanda: triceps — 9 cm, suprailiac — 13 cm, thigh — 19 cm
- Using Tables 3.2 and 3.3, determine the fitness category for David, Janessa, Shaun, and Amanda based on the body fats determined previously.

CARDIORESPIRATORY FITNESS: ESTIMATION FROM FIELD AND SUBMAXIMAL EXERCISE TESTS

- Jen is a 28-year-old businesswoman who has decided after being irregularly active since graduating college, it is time to "get back in shape." She goes to a local fitness center, and after all of her intake is completed, she comes back the next day to perform the Queens College step test, which yields a 15-second recovery HR of 36. Calculate and interpret Jen's cardiorespiratory fitness (CRF).
- Caleb decides to self-administer a 1-mile walk test to assess his fitness. He is 42-year-old, 6 ft. tall, and weighs 202 lb. Caleb exercises casually, usually involving strength training and inline skating. Caleb has an HR monitor and walks the 1 mile around a local high school track. Caleb's time to complete the mile walk was 10:45 seconds, and his peak HR was 148 bpm. Calculate Caleb's CRF, and interpret his fitness level.
- Candace is a 21-year-old college student who plays on the club rugby team. The rugby coach assesses the team's fitness using a submaximal cycle ergometer test. Candace's results show that stage 1 was at a work rate of $300 \text{ kg} \cdot \text{m}^{-1} \cdot \text{min}^{-1}$ and an HR of 121 bpm, and stage 2 was at a work rate of $450 \text{ kg} \cdot \text{m}^{-1} \cdot \text{min}^{-1}$ and an HR of 144 bpm. Calculate and interpret Candace's CRF. Using the de Souza equation, calculate Candace's CRF. How are the predicted $\dot{V}O_{2max}$ different using these two methods?
- Jackie, who weighs 150 lb, was given a submaximal cycle ergometer test using the YMCA protocol before starting an exercise program. The data from her test are as follows:
  - Age: 22 years
  - Weight: 150 lb
  - Stage 1: $150 \text{ kg} \cdot \text{m} \cdot \text{min}^{-1}$
  - Stage 2: $300 \text{ kg} \cdot \text{m} \cdot \text{min}^{-1}$; HR 132 bpm (steady state)
  - Stage 3: $450 \text{ kg} \cdot \text{m} \cdot \text{min}^{-1}$; HR 146 bpm (steady state)
    - Plot her data and determine her $\dot{V}O_{2max}$ in $\text{mL} \cdot \text{kg}^{-1} \cdot \text{min}^{-1}$.
- Six months later, she was tested again. Her data were as follows:
  - Age: 23 years
  - Weight: 145 lb
  - Stage 1: $150 \text{ kg} \cdot \text{m} \cdot \text{min}^{-1}$
  - Stage 2: $300 \text{ kg} \cdot \text{m} \cdot \text{min}^{-1}$; HR 126 bpm (steady state)
  - Stage 3: $450 \text{ kg} \cdot \text{m} \cdot \text{min}^{-1}$; HR 138 bpm (steady state)
    - Determine her $\dot{V}O_{2max}$ in $\text{mL} \cdot \text{kg}^{-1} \cdot \text{min}^{-1}$. How do you interpret her results in test #2 as compared to test #1 (consider $\dot{V}O_{2max}$ and her HR responses)?
- Sandy was also tested using the YMCA protocol. Her $\dot{V}O_{2max}$ in $\text{L} \cdot \text{min}^{-1}$ was estimated to be the same as Jackie's second test. However, her weight is 110 lb. What is her estimated $\dot{V}O_{2max}$ in $\text{mL} \cdot \text{kg}^{-1} \cdot \text{min}^{-1}$? How does this compare with Jackie's values? How do you explain the difference?

CARDIORESPIRATORY FITNESS: MAXIMAL EXERCISE TESTING

- Margo is a 42-year-old sedentary woman who went to her local fitness center to have her CRF measured. She chose to have a maximal exercise treadmill test done, but the testing supervisor selected the standard Bruce protocol for the test. Margo completed 6 minutes and 42 seconds on the treadmill before she signaled that she needed to stop. Her measured HR_{max} was 183 bpm, and her rating of perceived exertion (RPE) at test termination was 19; no other data were collected during the test. Determine Margo's $\dot{V}O_{2max}$ using both the nomogram in Figure 5.3 and the equation provided in Box 5.3. Compare the valued from the nomogram and the equation. Do the two $\dot{V}O_{2max}$ values match?
- Margo comes back to the fitness center 1 week later asking if she can do a different test to assess her $\dot{V}O_{2max}$ because she felt the Bruce protocol was too "hard." The testing supervisor suggests the modified Balke-Ware protocol, and Margo completes 13 minutes and again has an RPE of 19 at test termination. Determine Margo's $\dot{V}O_{2max}$ using the equation provided in Box 5.3. Do the two $\dot{V}O_{2max}$ values match? Was the $\dot{V}O_{2max}$ obtained with the modified Balke-Ware test similar to the $\dot{V}O_{2max}$ obtained with the Bruce protocol? If they are different, what might account for these differences?

MUSCULAR FITNESS

- The following case studies refer to the different needs in assessment between two separate 32-year-old women, Lauren, who weighs 124 lb, and her training partner Vanessa, who weighs 166 lb. Vanessa has considerable experience with fitness training, but Lauren is new to exercise.
  - Vanessa and Lauren each have different body weights and different levels of experience. Is it reasonable to use body weight during an assessment for both Lauren and Vanessa, why or why not? Does the level of experience matter when deciding to use body weight or not?
  - Considering the dynamic, static, and field tests available to assess muscular strength and muscular endurance, construct a list of tests that would be best suited for each Lauren and Vanessa, given their individual differences.
  - Both Lauren and Vanessa completed strength assessments of one repetition maximum (1-RM) for the bench press and were able to lift 125 lb on the bench press, whereas Lauren lifted 250 lb on the leg press compared to Vanessa's 305-lb leg press performance. Discuss how you would compare and interpret Lauren and Vanessa's muscular strength.

FLEXIBILITY

Terry is an office worker who has been working sitting in front of computers for 5 years. Since starting this job, she has seen a gradually increase in her weight, as a result of her sedentary lifestyle and hours in front of the computer. She contacts you to start an exercise program and is mostly interested in working on her flexibility. You perform a flexibility assessment, and you find the following:

Age: 35 years
Body weight: 70.5 kg
Height: 162.5 cm
Body composition: 38% body fat
Activity level: Light
Range of motion assessment

- Cervical flexion: 40 degrees, with slight discomfort
- Cervical extension: 45 degrees
- Lateral flexion: 40 degrees
- Lumbar spine: 2 in
- Lumbar extension: 0.5 in

Based on these values, how would you describe Terry's flexibility?
What kind of recommendations would you make for improvements?

Index